T0321659

ANIMAL ETHICS IN THE WILD

Animals, like humans, suffer and die from natural causes. This is particularly true of animals living in the wild, given their high exposure to, and low capacity to cope with, harmful natural processes. Most wild animals likely have short lives, full of suffering, usually ending in terrible deaths. This book argues that on the assumption that we have reasons to assist others in need, we should intervene in nature to prevent or reduce the harms wild animals suffer, provided that it is feasible and that the expected result is positive overall. It is of the utmost importance that academics from different disciplines as well as animal advocates begin to confront this issue. The more people concerned with wild animal suffering, the more probable it is that safe and effective solutions to the plight of wild animals will be implemented in the future.

CATIA FARIA is Assistant Professor of Applied Ethics at the Complutense University of Madrid and a founding member of the Centre for Animal Ethics at Pompeu Fabra University, Barcelona. She is the author of numerous articles and book chapters on wild animal suffering.

ANIMAL ETHICS IN THE WILD

Wild Animal Suffering and Intervention in Nature

CATIA FARIA

Complutense University of Madrid

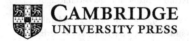
CAMBRIDGE
UNIVERSITY PRESS

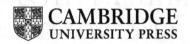

Shaftesbury Road, Cambridge CB2 8EA, United Kingdom

One Liberty Plaza, 20th Floor, New York, NY 10006, USA

477 Williamstown Road, Port Melbourne, VIC 3207, Australia

314–321, 3rd Floor, Plot 3, Splendor Forum, Jasola District Centre, New Delhi – 110025, India

103 Penang Road, #05–06/07, Visioncrest Commercial, Singapore 238467

Cambridge University Press is part of Cambridge University Press & Assessment, a department of the University of Cambridge.

We share the University's mission to contribute to society through the pursuit of education, learning and research at the highest international levels of excellence.

www.cambridge.org
Information on this title: www.cambridge.org/9781009113458

DOI: 10.1017/9781009119948

First published 2023
First paperback edition 2024

A catalogue record for this publication is available from the British Library

Library of Congress Cataloging-in-Publication data
NAMES: Faria, Catia, 1980– author.
TITLE: Animal ethics in the wild : wild animal suffering and intervention in nature / Catia Faria, Complutense University of Madrid.
DESCRIPTION: Cambridge, United Kingdom ; New York, NY : Cambridge University Press, 2023. | Includes bibliographical references and index.
IDENTIFIERS: LCCN 2022032385 (print) | LCCN 2022032386 (ebook) | ISBN 9781009100632 (hardback) | ISBN 9781009113458 (paperback) | ISBN 9781009119948 (epub)
SUBJECTS: LCSH: Animal welfare–Moral and ethical aspects. | Environmental ethics.
CLASSIFICATION: LCC HV4708 .F33 2023 (print) | LCC HV4708 (ebook) | DDC 179/.3–dc23/eng/
20220902
LC record available at https://lccn.loc.gov/2022032385
LC ebook record available at https://lccn.loc.gov/2022032386

ISBN   978-1-009-10063-2   Hardback
ISBN   978-1-009-11345-8   Paperback

Contents

Tables

Acknowledgments

I see this book as a collective endeavor. I would like to acknowledge the extraordinary encouragement, guidance, and support I have received from many people over the years. In particular, I express my gratitude to Núria Almiron, Paula Casal, and all my fellows at the UPF-Centre for Animal Ethics; and to Alexandra Abranches, João Rosas, and the rest of the colleagues who welcomed me at the Centre for Ethics, Politics and Society at the University of Minho. Special thanks are due to my friend, regular coauthor, and time traveler Eze Paez, who has accompanied me through the peaks and troughs of academia, of life, and of my own mind. I am also deeply grateful to Oscar Horta, my mentor and friend, for his help, vision, and commitment to what matters the most.

Many thanks are due as well to my chosen family, César, Marta, Momo, Nenna, and Rebk, without whose affective and social scaffolding I would simply not be alive today – Momo, in particular, brought beauty, energy, and the magic of connection to an otherwise rather dull existence; to my dear parents, Cândida and Albino, for their example of hard work, continuous support, and affection, and also for instilling in me, from a very young age, the quest for equality and social justice; to my sister Joana, who has taken on the difficult task of taking care of all of us, for her brilliance of mind and practical ability to solve problems in all dimensions of life; and to Aline, Fabiola, and Kris for their steady, genuine friendship. I am also forever indebted to Pablo (who made me happy), without whose *joy* this book would not have been started and, certainly, not finished. I further express my admiration and gratitude to all the people standing up for nonhuman animals within and outside academia and to all the philosophers who came before me.

Previous drafts of this book have greatly benefited from philosophical exchanges with multiple people, including Jeff McMahan, Alasdair Cochrane, Genoveva Martí, Peter Vallentyne, Kasper Lippert-Rasmussuen, Serena Olsaretti, Andrew Williams, and Clare Palmer. I am grateful to all of them. I also thank two anonymous reviewers for their helpful comments and for allowing me to clarify a number of problems, which, had they not been addressed, would have done little justice to the subject.

I would like to thank my editor at Cambridge University Press, Hilary Gaskin, for her consistent support, professionalism, and kindness, and also for accepting the delays resulting from two COVID-19 sick leaves. Nature is cruel, indeed. Or so this book argues.

I further thank Ruth Montiel Arias for providing us with one of her many wonderful photos to illustrate the cover of this book, and Victor Crespo for his help with the index.

Final thanks are due to Gerald, a decisive temporal part of my favorite four-dimensional object.

The research that led to this book received financial support from the Portuguese Foundation for Science and Technology, Grant: SFRH/BPD/116818/2016.

Introduction
Helping Animals

Nature, Mr. Allnut, is what we are put in this world to rise above.
Katherine Hepburn, in the *African Queen*

It seems to me that many theories of the universe may be dismissed at once, not as too good, but as too cosy, to be true. One feels sure that they could have arisen only among people living a peculiarly sheltered life at a peculiarly favourable period of the world's history. No theory need be seriously considered unless it recognises that the world has always been for most [humans] and all animals other than domestic pets a scene of desperate struggle in which great evils are suffered and inflicted.
C. D. Broad[1]

Comparisons, sad as they are, must be made to recognize where a great opportunity lies to prevent or mitigate suffering. The misery of animals in nature – which humans can do much to relieve – makes every other form of suffering pale in comparison. Mother Nature is so cruel to her children she makes Frank Perdue look like a saint.
Marc Sagoff[2]

This book relies on two main assumptions. Here is the first one: suffering is bad. Being burned alive or starving to death make you suffer. They feel bad. If you could do something to prevent bad things from happening, or otherwise alleviate their impact on individuals, without thereby bringing about more bad things in the world, and without jeopardizing anything of similar or greater importance, you ought to do it. This is the second assumption.

The moral case for helping others in need is very much premised on these two assumptions. It has been famously described in the literature by Peter Singer[3] in *The Drowning Child* experiment. Here is how it goes:

[1] Broad (1938, vol. 2, p. 774).
[2] Sagoff (1984, p. 303). Frank Perdue is the founder and CEO of Perdue Farms, one of the biggest chicken-producing corporations in the United States.
[3] See also Singer (1971) and Unger (1996).

I

To challenge my students to think about the ethics of what we owe to people in need, I ask them to imagine that their route to the university takes them past a shallow pond. One morning, I say to them, you notice a child has fallen in and appears to be drowning. To wade in and pull the child out would be easy but it will mean that you get your clothes wet and muddy, and by the time you go home and change you will have missed your first class. I then ask the students: do you have any obligation to rescue the child? Unanimously, the students say they do. The importance of saving a child so far outweighs the cost of getting one's clothes muddy and missing a class that they refuse to consider it any kind of excuse for not saving the child.[4]

Despite the students' reluctance to consider possible reasons for not saving the child, they (and the reader) are then asked to contemplate several variations on the original example that may change their intuitions. For instance, what if there are other bystanders who could also save the child, but nevertheless fail to do so? Do you still have reasons to pull the child out? The widespread intuition seems to be, again, that you ought to do it, no matter what others around you decide to do. But, then, Singer asks, would it make a difference if the child were not right in front of you but farther away, say, in a distant foreign country? Similarly, the common reaction is that, in itself, distance cannot ground a morally relevant difference between the two cases. Irrespective of distance or nationality, we should help that child in need.

The power of Singer's experiment is that it describes a real-world scenario. That is, in Singer's words, "we are all in that situation of the person passing the shallow pond: we can all save lives of people, both children and adults, who would otherwise die, and we can do so at a very small cost to us."[5] Therefore, we ought to do it, for instance, by donating to effective aid agencies. That seems right. To be sure, there are additional complications in the example. Yet, for present purposes, I will leave them aside.

Now consider a further variation on Singer's experiment. Imagine that instead of a human child, the individual in the pond is now a chimpanzee. We can call this *The Drowning Chimp*. Would *that* make a difference? One may confidently say that it would not. The fact that the child is *not human* is no reason for failing to help her. Appealing to species membership in order to justify responding differently in this case would be as unjustified as appealing to the child's sex or nationality in the previous one. For moral

---

[4] Singer (1997).   [5] Ibid.

purposes, they are all equally irrelevant criteria (for the time being, we can assume that this is indeed the case. I will provide support for this claim in Chapters 1 and 2).

As before, we can provide real-world analogs to this hypothetical scenario. Consider the following situation described by primatologist Jane Goodall:

> That polio outbreak in 1996 was one of the most traumatic times (. . .). It was just this one chimpanzee, Mr. McGregor, coming in, dragging with both paralyzed legs, and finally falling out of the tree and dislocating one arm (. . .). Gradually, other chimps appeared that we hadn't seen for a while, and they'd be dragging an arm or dragging a leg, or they never came back. It was an absolute terrible time. The doctor in Kigoma – the European doctor – knew there was an outbreak among people. He should have been administering the polio prevention drops. He hadn't done it. He should have (. . .). As soon as we realized, we immediately got the whole dose of the vaccine from Nairobi, and we would put the required number of drops into a banana (. . .). [I]t was a horrible, horrible time, and we lost many wonderful chimpanzees.[6]

Goodall had the vaccine. Her position was – in line with what we have seen before – that since she was capable of helping the sick chimpanzees and preventing many others from suffering the same fate, that is what she ought to do. In fact, as she states, "the European doctor" acted wrongly by failing to administer the polio prevention drops to the chimpanzees. Surely, Goodall did not believe that because they were not human beings, she did not have an obligation to help them. Rather, one might say, she had the belief that independently of considerations about species membership, their well-being and lives mattered to the extent that it provided her with compelling reasons to act on their behalf.

Many people would agree that Goodall did the right thing, while the European doctor acted wrongly. But then, again, it cannot make a difference whether the chimpanzee is right in front of you or farther away – for example, suffering and struggling in the wild. Distance and geographical situation are not, in themselves, morally relevant criteria. Thus, they cannot justify different responses in cases that are similar in all the important respects.

Yet some might object that Singer's and Goodall's are not relevantly analogous cases and thus do not allow us to infer the same conclusion. First, while in *The Drowning Child* we are all in a position to prevent or

---

[6] Academy of Achievement (2009). See also Goodall (1986).

alleviate some very bad things from happening to individuals in need, it is not the case that we are in a similarly suitable position regarding animals that suffer in the wild. Of course, not everyone is, as Jane Goodall, *in* the wild. Furthermore, there are not – or rather there are not as many[7] – aid agencies for wild animals. So, it could be argued, in the case of wild animals, the distance factor constitutes an insurmountable difficulty. Then, it might be added, perhaps no such agencies exist precisely because there is no need for that aid. While it is beyond any reasonable doubt that *these* particular animals are suffering and in need, these conditions are not representative of how animals fare in nature. Usually, wild animals live fairly well. Thus, it might be concluded, whereas there are indeed many distant human beings in need, and we therefore have an obligation to help them, often the best we can do for the majority of wild animals is just "to leave them alone."

This book is partly motivated by the aim to show that this is not the case. As a matter of fact, there are strong reasons to believe that the last objection is largely based on an idealized view of wild animals' lives. I will call this *the idyllic view of nature*.

One might distinguish between a strong and a weak version of the idyllic view as follows:

> *The strong idyllic view of nature:* the claim that wild animals typically have highly net positive lives.
> *The weak idyllic view of nature:* the claim that wild animals typically have good lives.

Although some may endorse the strong thesis, it is sufficient to consider the weaker thesis for the purposes of this analysis. I will show that we have reasons to believe that the weak idyllic view of nature is false, which entails a fortiori that the strong version of the view is so as well. A majority of wild animals *probably* have lives of intense suffering and a premature death. Additionally, whatever the truth about the predominance of suffering in nature, it is still the case that many wild animals experience a tremendous amount of suffering in their lives. Or so I will argue.

If the idyllic view is false, then we have as much reason to extrapolate from helping a particular chimpanzee in need to helping other wild animals in similar circumstances as we had to extend our positive obligations to help the drowning human child to help distant human beings in need. Of course, one might say, it would still have to be shown that in

---

[7] The Gorilla Doctors (www.gorilladoctors.org) constitutes a salient example.

both cases we are in an equally suitable position to help. For the moment, however, let us just proceed by formulating our problem in the following way:

> *The problem of wild animal suffering and intervention in nature*: ought we to prevent, or alleviate, the harms wild animals suffer in the wild?

The problem of wild animal suffering and intervention in nature has been, until some years ago, almost completely absent from the literature. Debates in animal ethics have predominantly focused on the reasons we may have to refrain from harming animals that are currently under human control.[8] There are apparently good reasons for this. Human action causes significant harm to an appalling number of animals that come into existence only to experience the daily suffering and the excruciating deaths associated with systemic animal exploitation.[9] If animal well-being is morally relevant and animals are made to suffer and killed while we could otherwise prevent it, then we ought to stop doing so.

In contrast, the situation of animals in the wild has not been seen as problematic. As a matter of fact, the belief that animal well-being is morally relevant has often been combined with the belief in a strong obligation of non-intervention in the wild – in turn, usually grounded, to a greater or lesser extent, on the aforementioned idyllic view of nature.[10]

Until very recently, few philosophers had challenged the compatibility of such beliefs and addressed the moral problem of wild animal suffering and intervention in nature. Some of them have done this by focusing on the moral problem of predation,[11] that is, the discussion about our reasons to intervene in the wild to prevent or reduce the harms inflicted on wild animals by their predators.

---

[8] See, for instance, Ryder (1975); Singer (2009 [1974]); Regan (1975, 2004 [1983]); LaFollette and Shanks (1996); Spiegel (1988); Fox (1999); Francione (2000, 2008); Cavalieri (2001); Cohen and Regan (2001); Nobis (2002); Rowlands (2002); Dunayer (2004); Sapontzis (ed.) (2004); Donaldson and Kymlicka (2011a); McPherson (2014); Bruers (2015).

[9] It is estimated that over sixty billion land animals and one to three trillion marine animals are bred or captured and brutally killed every year so that they can be converted into food products and clothing. Many more millions of animals are killed annually in worldwide experiments, after enduring painful and distressful experiences, such as incarceration and vivisection. Many others are in agony or desolation, confined, forced – and often killed – to entertain human populations in a wide array of circumstances. See FAO – Food and Agriculture Organization of the United Nations (2019); Mood and Brooke (2012); fishcount.org.uk (2012).

[10] See, for instance, Regan (2004 [1983]); Clark. (1977); Benton (1993); Gaard (ed.) (1993); Adams and Donovan (eds.) (1995, 2007); Donovan and Adams (eds.) (1996); Francione (2000); Dunayer (2004); Balcombe (2006); Donaldson and Kymlicka (2011a); Hadley (2015).

[11] Sapontzis (1984, 1987); Everett (2001); Cowen (2003); Fink (2005); McMahan (2010a, 2010b, 2015); Ebert and Machan (2012); Bramble (2021); Monsó (2021).

However, although it is the case that many wild animals are severely harmed by predatory activity, there are further causes of wild animal suffering in nature. Predation-induced harms only account for a fraction of the harms wild animals suffer. Notwithstanding that, it is true that many of the conclusions reached through investigating the moral problem of predation can be expanded to include other causes of wild animal suffering.[12]

Awareness about other forms of wild animal suffering, and especially by how they are determined by population ecology, has been triggered by the crucial work of Yew-Kwang Ng.[13] He claimed that the dynamics of animal populations in nature generates disvalue from the point of view of the individuals involved for the sake of natural processes. An increasing number of animal ethicists have been following the path opened by Ng's work and have offered more sustained philosophical arguments about the implications of accepting the magnitude of the disvalue that exists in nature. Others have also considered whether we should aid wild animals without necessarily assuming that natural disvalue is so high.[14]

Notwithstanding this, objections to aiding animals in nature based on a "laissez-faire intuition" according to which we should let nature be are still prevalent in the literature. Some of them are put forward by appealing to the nonexistence of morally relevant entanglements between human beings and wild animals in order to justify simply letting them be.[15] Others, while challenging the more traditional approaches to the wild as a "flat moral landscape ," have nevertheless been reluctant to accept more pervasive interventions in nature for the sake of wild animals. According to these authors, because wild animals are part of separate and sovereign "communities ," there is an obligation of non-interference, which implies a duty to preserve the ecosystems they inhabit.[16] This book will address these views and consider whether they are sound.

Another way in which intervention to aid wild animals may be opposed is by claiming that it conflicts with environmentalist aims. In fact, the relatively scarce work on wild animal suffering must be clearly demarcated

---

[12] Faria (2015).
[13] Ng (1995). Later popularized by Tomasik (2015a [2009]) and Horta (2010a, 2015).
[14] See Kirkwood and Sainsbury (1996); Bovenkerk et al. (2003); Clarke and Ng (2006); Hadley (2006); Morris and Thornhill (2006); Nussbaum (2006); Horta (2010a, 2015, 2017); Donaldson and Kymlicka (2011a); Dorado (2015); Faria and Paez (2015); Pearce (2015); Torres (2015); Faria (2018); Cochrane (2018); Faria and Horta (2019); Groff and Ng (2019); Johannsen (2020). This debate was pioneered by Victorian vegan avant la lettre and animal advocate Lewis Gompertz (1997 [1824]).
[15] Palmer (2010).   [16] Donaldson and Kymlicka (2011a).

from the extensive literature in environmental ethics, which endorses the moral considerability of other nonhuman contents of the natural world, such as species or ecosystems. The profound axiological and normative discrepancies between the main views in animal and environmental ethics have been conclusively established in the literature.[17] This book will not focus on such discrepancies but will address some of these environmentalist positions insofar as they are used as part of the case against intervention in the wild.

Animal Ethics in the Wild

We might think that, even if the problem of wild animal suffering and intervention in nature has been traditionally neglected, that should not worry us since it is not a very important problem. However, this is a moral issue that may seriously affect a great number of individuals. The number of animals in the wild vastly surpasses the number of animals under human control.[18] Thus, considering both the work that needs to be done and the billions that can benefit from it, a few other issues may be considered, on the same criteria, more important.[19]

I proceed as follows. I start by examining two traditional debates in animal ethics: Chapter 1 discusses the reasons why nonhuman animals are morally considerable, and Chapter 2 explains the concept and justification of speciesism. I will work under the assumption that, other things being equal, the conclusions reached throughout these chapters will apply similarly both to nonhuman animals under human control and nonhuman animals living in the wild. In Chapter 3 , I examine the empirical evidence about wild animal suffering – in particular, data from population dynamics – in order to determine the magnitude of the problem. I will then assess the extent to which the available evidence, together with the normative views defended in the previous two chapters, gives us reasons to intervene in nature on behalf of wild animals.

[17] See, for instance, Callicott (1980); Sagoff (1984); Hargrove (ed.) (1992); Crisp (1998), Faria and Paez (2019).

[18] In a rough estimate, the number of sentient animals living in the wild could rise to 10^{21} or 10^{22} according to Tomasik (2015a [2009]).

[19] Peter Singer himself has suggested that this is one of the most pressing moral issues and encouraged moral philosophers to do research on it, and others to find ways that will make it increasingly more feasible to help animals in the wild, for instance, at the International Conference on Ethics at the University of Porto, June 21, 2019.

Having cleared the ground, both philosophically and empirically, I provisionally claim that there are decisive reasons to aid animals in nature. The main goal of this book is not to elaborate a complete argument for intervention in nature from one or several normative perspectives. Instead, it presents a very broad and minimal case for reducing wild animal suffering and then focuses on what I consider to be the most salient objections that might be raised against it. The minimal case for intervention in nature is based primarily on a series of plausible moral and factual claims about wild animal suffering. It is compatible with most important ethical theories (or, at least, with those that accept the existence of positive obligations) and can therefore – or so I hope – attract wide support. I will deal with this latter point in the conclusion of the book.

Since the number of possible objections to this view is very large, it was necessary to develop a taxonomy to organize them. I elaborate on Albert O. Hirschman's classification of the arguments against social progress (the arguments from perversity, futility, and jeopardy) in *The Rhetoric of Reaction*.[20] In Chapter 4 , I then discuss perversity and futility objections to intervention, while in chapter 5 I analyze jeopardy objections. Three types of objections to intervention, however, do not sit comfortably in Hirschman's taxonomy and are discussed in three separate chapters. In Chapter 6 , I debate relational objections, while in Chapter 7 I focus on what one may term priority objections. Finally, Chapter 8 deals with objections that arise from tractability concerns.

I conclude that if it is feasible to prevent or alleviate wild animal suffering by intervening in nature, without thereby bringing about an expected worse state of affairs for the individuals affected, we ought to do it. Moreover, for those interventions currently infeasible, we should put ourselves in a position to achieve them, both individually and collectively.

Finally, "nonhuman animals that live in nature" is quite the cumbersome locution. It would be awkward to employ it every time I refer to the individuals I am discussing. Thus, I will sometimes refer to them, loosely and variously, as "animals in nature ," "animals in the wild," or even "wild animals ." I am aware, however, that the terms are not strictly speaking co-extensive. Worse still, referring to wild animals may suggest that they are fierce or aggressive. Nevertheless, my use of this term is to be understood without that particular connotation. Furthermore, also for linguistic economy, I will often use simply "animals" to refer to nonhuman animals. Finally, someone may wonder why not simply use the expression "free-living

[20] Hirschman (1991).

animals," now so much in vogue. My answer is that the expression should be avoided inasmuch as it remains an open question whether wild animals are free at all.[21] Moreover, unless there is evidence of an individual's self-identified pronoun, I will use "they" as a generic third-person singular pronoun to refer to any individual (human and nonhuman) whose gender is unknown or irrelevant to the context of the usage.[22]

---

[21] For the view that wild animals are socially, or politically, unfree, see, for instance, Paez (2021).

[22] See APA Style and Grammar Guidelines from the American Psychological Association (2020).

CHAPTER I

Moral Considerability

In this chapter, I claim that wild animals are morally considerable beings. I argue that because nonhuman animals are sentient, they have a well-being of their own – a necessary and sufficient condition for having moral consideration. I further argue that nonhuman animals' interest in avoiding suffering is morally relevant and that taking this interest into account may require different courses of action from moral agents. Finally, I assess whether (and to what extent), under certain theoretical assumptions, death may be bad for nonhuman animals.

1.1   Moral Considerability Explained

Arguments about the moral considerability of nonhuman animals (i.e., about whether animals are the sort of entities that should be taken into account in our moral deliberation) usually proceed as follows:

(i)   A certain attribute (e.g., a capacity) x bestows moral considerability.
(ii) Animal P possesses x.
(iii) Therefore, P is morally considerable.

The attribute possessed by many animals, which is usually considered relevant for moral considerability in the animal ethics literature, is *sentience*. By "sentience" I will refer here to the capacity to have conscious experiences of positive or negative valence. Even if it is still a matter of contention whether some animals do have such capacity, it is well beyond any reasonable doubt that many of them do.[1] The scientific consensus is now that vertebrates and octopuses are sentient, whereas the jury is still out

---

[1] See, for instance, Dawkins (2012 [1980]); Griffin (1981, 1992); Rollin (1989); Smith (1991); Sandøe and Simonsen (1992); De Grazia (1996); Allen and Bekoff (1997); Mather (2001); Gregory (2004); Eaton et al. (2006); Haynes (2008); Braithwaite (2010); Broom (2014).

regarding other invertebrates and we have various degrees of evidence regarding different taxa.[2]

Although far from uncontroversial, this view nowadays enjoys wide acceptance. Many authors have argued for the moral relevance of the capacity for positive and negative conscious experiences, claiming it is sufficient for an individual to have a well-being of their own.[3] From this position, these writers have often arrived at a series of conclusions about the unjustified character of the human exploitation of nonhuman animals. Nevertheless, they have seldom explored the implications that accepting sentience as sufficient for moral considerability has for those animals that live in the wild. Particularly, they have rarely approached the problem of whether we should intervene in nature to help them when they are in need.

The aim of this book is to examine whether these implications indeed follow for nonhumans living in the wild once we accept this premise. It lies beyond the scope of this book to provide a complete argument about the relevance of sentience for moral considerability.[4] My point of departure, then, shall consist in accepting the view that if an individual has a well-being of their own, then they are morally considerable. Most of us would agree that having a well-being is a condition satisfied by most nonhuman animals, given that they can have positive and negative experiences.[5] Certainly, some have denied this by claiming that nonhuman animals are automata without mental states, but nowadays few philosophers still agree with such a view. Because it is sufficiently uncontroversial, in this book I will not argue either for the claim that there are animals that are

---

[2] See, for instance, Low et al. (2012); Birch (2020). See also Rethink Priorities (2020) as a remarkable example of an NGO that takes the topic very seriously and attempts to assign degrees of credence to the sentience of different invertebrates.

[3] See, for instance, Gompertz (1997 [1824]); Salt (1980 [1892]); Nelson (1956); Godlovitch (1971); Godlovitch et al. (1971); Singer (2009 [1974], 2011 [1979]); Ryder (1975); Regan (1975, 2004 [1983]); Clark (1977); Rollin (1981); Sapontzis (1987); Rachels (1990); Pluhar (1995); Dombrowski (1996); LaFollette and Shanks (1996); Bernstein (1998, 2015); Rowlands (1998); Francione (2000, 2008); Cavalieri (2001); Dunayer (2004); Garner (2005); Korsgaard (2005); Aaltola (2012).

[4] I will attempt to sketch out the argument very briefly. Our criteria of moral considerability should be grounded on whatever attributes are relevant for the purposes of moral decision-making. When engaged in moral reasoning affecting different individuals, an agent deliberates about which of the different available courses of action to undertake, given (at least in part) how they affect themselves and other individuals. The fact that a being can be affected by a certain action or event and, thereby, be harmed or benefited by it is, therefore, sufficient grounds for moral considerability. Those beings who can be harmed or benefited by agents are those who have a well-being of their own. Thus, moral considerability should be granted to those entities who can have a well-being of their own. For a detailed discussion, see Horta (2018).

[5] Bernstein (1998, p. 16).

sentient. As stated, my aim in this work is to examine what follows if we accept this, together with other plausible views.

Therefore, it can hardly be claimed that many nonhuman animals are not morally considerable by claiming that they are not sentient. A different way to do so, however, would be to claim that, even if many nonhuman animals are sentient, they do not have a well-being of their own. I will examine this view in the following section.

1.2 Nonhuman Well-Being

The best way to proceed in order to examine whether nonhuman animals have a well-being of their own seems to be by considering, first, what the most accepted accounts of well-being claim it encompasses. That will enable us, later, to determine whether nonhuman animals can indeed possess well-being. According to the most widespread classification,[6] there are three such accounts: hedonism (also called experientialism or mental state welfarism),[7] the desire-based theory (also known as desire satisfactionism),[8] and the objective list theory.[9] I will now discuss what each of these views claims, as well as their implications for nonhuman animals in light of the criterion for moral considerability presented above.

From a hedonist perspective, an experience of pleasure – generated, say, by P satisfying an intense thirst – contributes to P's well-being, whereas an experience of intense suffering – caused, for instance, by an illness – detracts from it.[10] Thus, P has an interest in having their thirst satisfied and an interest in avoiding pain and other negative experiences. P is, therefore, harmed when their interests in having positive experiences and in avoiding adverse ones are disregarded, so that either P is led to suffer from negative experiences or they are deprived of positive experiences they might otherwise have had. Conversely, P is benefited when these interests are satisfied.

---

[6] Parfit (1984, pp. 493–501).

[7] Sumner (1996); Feldman (2004). Strictly speaking, not all forms of experimentalism are hedonist. For instance, a position that valued the variety of experiences would not qualify as hedonist. For simplicity, though, I will refer to the general account as "hedonism."

[8] Griffin (1986); Heathwood (2006).   [9] Hurka (1993); Nussbaum (2006).

[10] I shall use the term "suffering" in its inclusive usage so as to denote any negative affective state that includes an unpleasant consciousness or feeling. Suffering and its positive counterpart – pleasure (or happiness) – conjointly comprise the full valence of affective experience. Moreover, a negative axiology, although it does not need to deny that feel-good mental states exist, would claim that they have no positive moral value. See Gloor (2019 [2016]).

Now suppose we accept the aforementioned assumption that the possession of a capacity to have a well-being suffices for moral considerability. If hedonism is right and the only thing that matters for well-being is the value of experiences, then all beings with the capacity for having such experiences are morally considerable. If we have reasons not to harm, as well as reasons to benefit, individuals with a well-being of their own, nonhuman animals' interests in having positive experiences and in avoiding negative ones give us reasons for acting on their behalf.

An alternative account of well-being, the desire-based theory, would claim that what contributes to an individual's well-being is how the said individual's desires are satisfied and frustrated, rather than their positively or negatively valenced experiences. Suppose that P desires that p. According to this theory, P has an interest that their desire be satisfied, as well as an interest in avoiding the frustration of that desire, independently of the conduciveness of their desires to positive or negative experiences regarding p. Preventing P from fulfilling their desire that p thus harms them whereas satisfying P's desire that p benefits them.[11]

Some might say that we can escape bestowing moral consideration to nonhuman animals if we believe that a desire-based theory such as this offers a more compelling account than hedonism of what makes an individual's life go well or badly. The reason would be that the formation of desires allegedly requires a more sophisticated cognitive capacity than mere sentient experience. Thus, so the argument goes, by lacking the relevant desire formation capacity, merely sentient beings (e.g., many nonhuman animals but also human infants) would not have a well-being of their own. Only those who do have those sophisticated capacities would. However, this seems counterintuitive. One may plausibly ask,

> Assuming one was convinced of an infant's incapability of forming desires, would a mother be acting irrationally by requesting anaesthesia for her daughter during an operation? Surely, we are diminishing the welfare of a dog by mercilessly beating it [*sic*], even if the dog is incapable of desiring that the beating be stopped.[12]

The point is that if an individual is in great pain or in any other aversive state, it seems implausible to claim that because they lack the cognitive endowment necessary to form desires about their own subjective experience, their life is not going badly for them.

---

[11] In antifrustrationist versions of this view, frustrated desires are harmful, whereas satisfied desires are neutral, and thus equivalent to having no desires. See Fehige (1998).

[12] Bernstein (1998, p. 77).

Nonetheless, it is possible to account for this within a desire-based theory. One way to do so would be to claim that desires must be understood counterfactually. That is, desires whose satisfaction counts for an individual's well-being are not necessarily those they actually have but those that they would have with the relevant information and under certain specified conditions of rational reflection.[13] Of course, if that is so, the same applies to both human and nonhuman sentient beings since there is, in principle, nothing that prevents the same counterfactual situation from obtaining in either case.

In addition, there is a more straightforward way in which desire satisfactionists can deny that one needs to have complex cognitive abilities in order to form the appropriate sort of desires. They can argue that if an individual has a certain negative experience, then that entails that such an individual will develop a desire against having that experience. Some have even argued that it is the fact that such a desire is formed that bestows negative valence to an experience.[14] If one accepts this view, then it must be concluded that the domain of the beings that can be benefited or harmed according to a desire-based account will, at least, include[15] the domain that would be drawn by those who claim that only mental states can be valuable or disvaluable.

Therefore, each of these two ways allows us to conclude that sentient nonhuman animals can have a well-being of their own. Again, if that is what is necessary for moral consideration, then, according to desire-satisfactionist theories, nonhuman animals are morally considerable.

Finally, an objective list account of well-being would consider that well-being is determined by the presence or absence of certain elements that are objectively good or bad, in a mind-independent way, for the individuals who are capable of accessing them. Thus, if P has an interest in x, then that would be so independently of x generating any positive or negative experience for P or x being the object of P's desire. The mere presence or absence of x would be what harms or benefits P. Something can be of interest to an individual even if it does not generate any valenced state.

Some may claim that on the best objective list account of well-being there are no objective goods that are present in the lives of nonhuman animals. Likewise, they could claim that there are no objective bads in

---

[13] Singer (2011 [1979]); de Lazari-Radek and Singer (2014, pp. 225–227).

[14] See Sidgwick (1996 [1874]).

[15] Just to be safe, I do not rule out the possibility of an artificial agent with valenced states, the grounds of which valence are desires all the way down, without there being a fundamental level of feeling-based valence.

their lives either that we might have reason to prevent from happening. This view is, however, very difficult to accept. The claim that it is not bad for an animal in intense pain to suffer appears to be highly implausible.[16] In addition, this view also has counterintuitive consequences for the human case since it implies that there are no objective goods or bads in a life of a human being with similar psychological capacities. If some item in the objective list is valuable for an individual, then it must be so as well for others who can enjoy it. For instance, if, as an objective list theorist might claim, knowledge is good for you, then it seems difficult to deny that it can be good for me too. Accordingly, if suffering is in itself bad for a human being, it must be bad also for other beings who can experience it. Thus, it must be bad for nonhuman animals.

For that not to be the case, it should be for reasons different from the nature of suffering itself. Some may argue that suffering is bad for a human being, but for a nonhuman animal, because only the former has certain complex cognitive capacities. Yet this contradicts the usual view about why suffering is bad. Suffering (as we experience it when we feel extreme pain) seems to be bad for us simply because of how it feels. We do not believe that, if our cognitive capacities were higher, the pain of a burn would be worse for us. Moreover, if pain was bad for us because of our cognitive capacities, we would have to reject the assumption presented before that whether a certain item in the objective list is good or bad for someone depends on the capacity an individual has to possess it. Denying that, however, seems to be unjustified.

According to this, it seems that any plausible version of the objective list theory must include basic hedonic experiences at least as part of what is objectively good (or bad). According to these positions, therefore, sentient nonhuman animals have a well-being of their own. If this is what matters in order to be morally considerable, then again sentient nonhuman animals will be so.

To conclude, as Parfit famously put it,

> These three theories partly overlap. On all these theories, happiness and pleasure are at least part of what makes our lives go better for us, and misery and pain are at least part of what makes our lives go worse. These claims would be made by any plausible Objective List Theory. And they are implied by all versions of the Desire-Fulfilment theory. On all theories, the Hedonistic Theory is at least part of the truth.[17]

---

[16] See, for instance, Sapontzis (1987); Nussbaum (2006).   [17] Parfit (1984, p. 4).

Accordingly, on any plausible account of well-being, sentient nonhuman animals are individuals with a well-being of their own that can be harmed or benefited by our actions. First, either hedonic experiences are all that matter or they are at least part of what is objectively good. In either case, nonhuman positive and negative hedonic experiences necessarily matter too. Second, if what matters instead is how individual desires are fulfilled, then on the most plausible accounts of desires positive and negative hedonic experiences give rise to desires for and against their presence that can be fulfilled or thwarted.

This implies that sentience is a necessary and sufficient condition for any individual P to have a well-being. Sentience is defined as the capacity for valenced mental states. It is therefore a precondition for possessing such states, such as suffering and enjoyment. Thus, if a being is sentient, they can be affected positively or negatively by events.

Many nonhuman animals satisfy this condition. They can suffer and enjoy what occurs to them and hence their lives can go well or badly insofar as their interests are negatively or positively affected.

Given all this, if we accept the assumption pointed out above that those beings that have a well-being must be morally considerable, there are strong reasons to conclude that sentient animals should be morally considerable individuals. The question that may now arise is the *extent* to which their well-being matters. This will be assessed in the following sections.

1.3   Equal Consideration

The principle of equal consideration states that equal interests of different individuals count the same, regardless of the identity of those individuals. Yet, in order to understand this claim, one must first characterize what an interest is. The term "interests" can actually be understood in several different ways. But here I will simply employ it according to its widespread usage in the animal ethics literature. In that sense, P has an interest in x if and only if x contributes to P's well-being.[18] Accordingly, a being has an interest in what contributes to their well-being and in avoiding what detracts from it. Of course, the answer to what would be most in an individual's interests will depend on the theory of well-being one endorses.

What the principle of equal consideration states is that if a being has an interest in not suffering, their suffering must be accounted for just as it

---

[18] See Feinberg (1980).

would if it were the equal suffering of another individual. Two equal interests are two interests that are comparatively equally important to those who have them. Accordingly, an equal interest in not suffering is an interest of the same weight, corresponding to an instance of suffering of an equivalent intensity and duration. All things being equal, any change in the weight of an interest in not suffering obtains just in case there is a change in the intensity or the duration of the suffering experienced. Thus, if P and Q instantiate equally intense suffering and for an equally long time, P and Q have equal interests in not suffering. The principle of equal consideration claims that, if this is so, then P's and Q's interests in not suffering should have the same weight in moral deliberation. In other words, it claims that those interests provide us with equally strong reasons for action.

An important implication of this principle is that independently of the species to which P and Q belong, their equal interests should be equally considered. Thus, giving greater weight to the similar interests of Q (e.g., human) over P (e.g., nonhuman) would be unjustified.

Of course, one may wonder about the reasons for accepting this principle. The first reason is that it appears to be the default view on the consideration of individual interests. This is so because if we accept that the interests of all individuals matter, and we are not provided with any further reasons to take into account that may draw differences among them, it then seems that these interests must matter equally. If that were not the case, it would have to be because of other, additional reasons. Yet until those reasons were provided, and until they were verified as sound, we ought to conclude that equal interests count the same, given that we have the same reasons to consider them – that is, that they are all interests of some weight.

Some may dispute that the interests of humans and nonhuman animals should count the same. They may claim that when making interspecies comparisons of suffering, it is false that humans and other animals have an equal interest in not suffering. Due to human beings' higher cognitive capacities, so may the argument go, their suffering is much worse compared to that of nonhuman animals under similar circumstances. This objection, however, is controversial, and it also misses the point. Whether humans suffer more than nonhuman animals under similar circumstances is not something that affects the normative claim that, when humans suffer just as much as other animals, their suffering should count the same. The principle of equal consideration claims that equal interests count the same, not that unequal interests count the same.

Moreover, while there are circumstances in which humans do suffer more than nonhuman animals, the opposite can also be the case. Consider, for example, a hypothetical experiment on a human individual in which a significant amount of pain was inflicted on them over a long period of time. Insofar as the human being would be able to conceptualize the suffering inflicted upon them, the argument goes, their suffering would be worse than the suffering of an animal of another species undergoing the same experiment but lacking such capacity. Thus, the argument concludes, human interests in not suffering are stronger than nonhumans' and should thus be favored over the interests in not suffering of members of other species.

Yet the objection is misguided, as it has been successfully shown in the literature.[19] Possession of higher cognitive capacities does not necessarily lead to experiencing worse instances of suffering. In fact, it can have the opposite effect. As Rollin says,

> In terms of countering the pernicious moral power of the claim that animals can't anticipate and remember pain and that therefore their pain is insignificant, the most relevant point has little to do with the presence or absence of concepts. It comes rather from the following insight: That if animals are indeed, as the above argument suggests, inexorably locked into what is happening in the here and now, we are all the more obliged to try to relieve their suffering, since they themselves cannot look forward to or anticipate its cessation, or even remember, however dimly, its absence. If they are in pain, their whole universe is pain; there is no horizon; they *are* their pain. So, if the argument is indeed correct, then animal pain is terrible to contemplate, for the dark universe of animals logically cannot tolerate any glimmer of hope within its borders.[20]

The point can be pressed even further. Consider a slight qualification of the previous example. Imagine that the experiment is necessary to make the life of the affected individual worth living. While the individual with a higher cognitive apparatus would be able to understand the net value of the procedure, it would be impossible for the low-capacity individual to apprehend it, and thus their suffering would be comparatively much worse. Moreover, even if it were the case that high-capacity individuals had a stronger interest in not suffering than low-capacity individuals, the argument would still fail to show that *human* interests in not suffering are stronger than nonhuman ones since many human beings would also fail to

[19] For instance, Singer (2009 [1974]); Rollin (1981); Sapontzis (1987); Pluhar (1995); Bernstein (1998); Cavalieri (2001); Horta (2010b).
[20] Rollin (1989, p. 144).

exemplify the alleged relevant capacity (this will be discussed in more detail in Chapter 2). So, if our reasons to reduce someone's suffering depend on the weight of their suffering and not on their species, it is false that human interests in not suffering provide us with stronger reasons to prevent it than similar interests in not suffering of nonhuman individuals.

Nevertheless, as stated above, this is not to deny that satisfying the interest in not suffering of different individuals may require, sometimes, different actions from moral agents. In fact, when facing the same event, different individuals may not suffer equally. In that sense, the principle of equal consideration does not necessarily entail an obligation of equal treatment. For example, when punched with the same strength, a human baby and a human adult may experience a different intensity of suffering. Likewise, a similarly strong punch, when given to a piglet, may cause greater suffering than when given to an adult human being. Equal consideration of interests requires, then, accounting for such differences among individuals.

1.4 The Badness of Death

Thus far, it has been argued that if we accept that it is bad that nonhuman animals suffer, and that we have reasons to prevent this from happening, then, whenever we can, we should help them when they are in need. This is sufficient to build a positive case for aiding wild animals.

A different topic is whether nonhuman animals are harmed by death and whether, due to this, we should intervene to save their lives when possible. It is not really necessary to examine this problem in order to assess whether we should help animals in the wild since, as indicated, for this purpose it is enough to take their suffering into account. Nevertheless, it can be useful to proceed with such an examination. If nonhuman animals are harmed by death, then there will be further reasons to aid those animals whose lives are at risk, and these reasons should be added to those we already have to prevent their suffering.

As argued in the previous section, because human and nonhuman animals have an interest in not suffering, whenever death causes sentient beings to suffer to the same extent, it necessarily harms them equally. Yet the question we are asking here is a different one. It is not whether *painful* death harms nonhuman animals, but rather whether, independently of the suffering experienced at the moment of dying, animals are harmed by ceasing to exist.[21] For simplicity, I will henceforth use "death" to refer to death as such, independently of the suffering that may accompany it when it occurs.

This debate is independent of the one about what death consists in and the underlying ontological views about the persistence conditions over time of sentient individuals. In this section, I will put these ontological issues aside and focus exclusively on how to determine whether and to what extent death can be bad for nonhuman animals. In order to examine this problem, I will first assess a standard account of the harm of death, the one that claims that death is bad insofar as it deprives us of future goods.

a)   The Deprivation Account

There is widespread – even if not universal – agreement that if death is bad, then it is because of what it deprives us of. Since Thomas Nagel's influential article "Death,"[22] the Deprivation Account has now been established as the "orthodox view" about the badness of death.[23]

> *The Deprivation Account.* Death is bad for an individual because it deprives them of a further life that would have been good for them.

Death thus harms individuals because it takes away from them all the goods that life would contain if they had remained alive. One implication of this is that sometimes death may be good. This happens in those cases in which it deprives individuals of a life not worth living. For example, if by dying at a certain time someone is prevented from experiencing excruciating suffering over a period of 24 hours after which they would have died anyway, then compared to the remaining life they would otherwise have experienced, death was not bad for them. Another implication of this is that depending on the amount of good that a life might include, death can be more or less bad for individuals. Consider, for instance, the case of someone dying at 20 when they could have lived a good life until 80, and the death of someone dying at 80 that could have lived 5 more good years. While we could consider both deaths to be harmful, we would think of the

---

[21]   Singer (2011 [1979]); McMahan (2002); Višak (2013); Višak and Garner (2016).
[22]   Nagel (1970).
[23]   In present times, the Deprivation Account has been defended by Feldman (1992); Feit (2002); Bradley (2009). For objections to the Deprivation Account, see Epicurus (1964 [ca. 300 BC]); Silverstein (1980); Suits (2001). For a critical discussion of this view, see also McMahan (1988, 2002); Kamm (1993); French and Wettstein (eds.) (2000); Scarre (2007); Belshaw (2009); Luper (2009).

death of the twenty-year-old (compared with the future life they could have lived) as a greater misfortune since the eighty-year-old would have lost fewer years of life.[24]

Note that this account is not committed to any particular view about what makes a life go well or badly for someone. In fact, the Deprivation Account might be further completed with different axiological assumptions, such that

(i)   Death at t is bad for the individual P who dies if it deprives P of a future of net positive experiences (hedonism).

(ii) Death at t is bad for the individual P who dies if it deprives P of a future of net desire-fulfillment (desire-based theory).

(iii) Death at t is bad for the individual P who dies if it deprives P of a future containing a net amount of objectively good things (objective-list theory).

Thus, according to the Deprivation Account, in order to decide whether the death of an individual is bad for them, their actual level of well-being must be compared to the well-being they would have had if they remained alive. For example, suppose that Nico died at age 20. Let us assume, for simplicity, that the right theory of well-being is hedonism. The total sum of positive and negative experiences Nico suffered during their lifetime has a net positive amount of 250 units of well-being. Had they remained alive, they would have had 20 more good years and then suffered during their final 5 ones. Had they not died, their lifetime well-being would have been 450. Subtracting this value from their actual lifetime well-being level of 250 gives us −200. This is the disvalue of Nico dying at age 20 instead of at 45. We can thus consider that their death was very bad for them. If, however, the last years of Nico's life had been spent in misery, their death at 20 instead of at 45 would have been good for them.

Now, if we accept that the Deprivation Account offers an adequate explanation of why the death of human beings might be a bad thing for them, we might then ask whether under the same assumption death may be bad for nonhuman animals as well. Since the death of nonhuman animals also involves the deprivation of the goods they might have otherwise enjoyed if they had not died, it seems to follow that death harms them too. Thus, all things being equal, they have an interest in not being harmed, by continuing to live.

---

[24] According to a more radical, egalitarian, deprivationist view, the harm of death grows in a way inversely proportional to how much one has lived in the past. See Cavalieri (2001).

There have been, however, different attempts to dispute this implication. The first one, which assumes a desire-based view, consists in denying that death is bad for nonhuman animals since they cannot be attributed the relevant desire, which is the desire to continue to live. The second attempt consists in claiming that while it is true that death deprives nonhuman animals of their future life, what they lose in dying must be discounted by some other variable.

b) The Attribution of Desires

As previously mentioned, from a desire-based view, death can be bad for an individual insofar as it deprives them of a future of net desire-fulfillment. Some desire satisfactionists, however, understand differently the way in which death can be harmful. According to Ruth Cigman, for instance, death is harmful just in case it frustrates some desires we now have.[25] This can happen in two ways:

(i)   P can be harmed by death if, and only if, P has an actual desire to live, which presupposes the capacity to formulate certain relevant concepts (such as the concept of themselves as a temporally extended individual).

Or,

(ii)   P can be harmed by death if, and only if, P has long-term future-oriented desires for whose satisfaction continuing to live is instrumentally necessary (e.g., having a career).

Either of these views requires a strong cognitive apparatus for the formation of a desire to live, which most animals fail to possess (e.g., self-awareness). Only long-term future-oriented individuals, with a capacity to see themselves as extended over time, can have a desire to continue to live and can have long-term future-oriented desires. Only they, these views conclude, can be harmed by death, which thwarts those desires. Allegedly, most humans can project themselves to the far future, covering the whole extent of their lives. Therefore, death would deprive them of that whole future. On the contrary, most nonhuman animals, by lacking the necessary psychological capacities to harbor the relevant desires, cannot be harmed by death. Hence, they have no interest in continuing to live that gives us reasons against killing them or preventing them from dying.

[25] Cigman (1980).

Against these views, what the desire-fulfillment version of the Deprivation Account implies, as we saw above, is that death harms an individual merely if it deprives them of a future of net desire-fulfillment. For that to be possible, the only condition that needs to obtain is the following one:

(iii)   P can be harmed by death if P has short-term future-oriented desires for whose satisfaction continuing to live is instrumentally necessary (e.g., eating, resting, avoiding suffering . . .).

Unlike the previous criteria, this one seems to be satisfied not only by humans but also by other animals. There seems to be extremely strong evidence that many nonhuman animals qualify for having the relevant desires according to (iii). Although controversial, this view is capable of accommodating strong intuitions about the desire to continue to live of human beings that would also fail to qualify for the relevant desire on (i) and (ii). That would be the case, for example, of human beings lacking complex cognitive capacities to form a desire to live or humans lacking self-chosen future projects or goals. Under (i) and (ii), these human beings would simply lack an interest in continuing to live. According to (iii), however, their short-term desires would sufficiently ground an interest in remaining alive.

Against this view, it could be argued that even if we accept that having short-term desires is sufficient to have an interest in living, the strength of that interest would still be proportional to how far in time one can picture future life events that concern them. The implication of this would be that the interest in not dying of an individual with a similarly valuable future, but with lesser capacity to project themselves into the future, would be less weighty than the interest of an individual who can be attributed a desire to live that covers their whole future. Individuals with no capacity to project themselves into the future would still not qualify for having the relevant desire. All else being equal, the strength of our reasons to prevent the frustration of such an interest would therefore have to be correspondingly adjusted. This would be a combination of the Deprivation Account of the Badness of Death and the claim that death is harmful as long as we have long-term future-oriented desires. Nevertheless, if, as argued, the Deprivation Account adequately explains why death is a harm, we do not need to accept such a view.

Another objection would consist in claiming that only those beings with complex intellectual capacities can form desires. However, as previously mentioned, on the most plausible versions of the desire-based view, this is not so. We can thus conclude that all beings with a capacity for positive and negative experiences can be said to have desires. This conclusion follows clearly if we assume the view that whenever we have a positive or negative experience, we automatically develop a preference for and against it. This view implies that all beings who can have a positive experience will have a satisfied preference whenever such a benefit occurs. If this is so, that means that such a being will satisfy the condition of having short-term desires that the Deprivation Account of the Badness of Death requires for someone to be harmed by dying.

Consider now the view that the desires we should care about are not those that individuals actually have but those that they would have formed under ideal conditions of deliberation. These desires would thus exist in a non-actual possible world. One could oppose this by claiming that nonhuman animals are harmed by death by saying that we must only care about ideal desires that exist in possible worlds that are closest to ours in some respect. Some believe[26] that those possible worlds are the ones in which the individual in question has psychological capacities similar to those they possess in the actual world. That would exclude the worlds in which nonhuman individuals have the necessary capacities to desire to live. It is unclear, however, how this restriction may be justified.

The appeal of an ideal version of the desire-based view, as opposed to an actual desire version, is that it tells us to be concerned for the desires an individual would have if they possessed all the relevant information and conducted a faultless reasoning. On the view we are considering here, we are thereby excluding from our consideration those possible worlds in which a sentient individual possesses the psychological capacities that would allow them to deliberate in that way. Thus, we are settling for desires which, in the case of beings with complex cognitive capacities, we would not consider as determinant of the interests of individuals, as given by their well-being.

There is a straightforward way, then, in which an appeal to ideal desires leads us to conclude that it is justified to attribute a desire to live to any sentient individual with a net valuable future. Actually, it follows that it would be unjustified not to do so. This is because that is a desire which that individual would actually entertain if they had all the information and deliberated under ideal conditions. In such a version of the desire-based view, the interest in continuing to live of a nonhuman sentient is as strong

---

[26] For instance, Singer (2011 [1979]).

as the interest in continuing to live of a cognitively complex human with a similarly worthy future.

Therefore, there are adequately plausible versions of the desire-based view in which death may harm nonhumans. These accounts can grant that death harms nonhumans as much as it harms humans, depending on the future they are deprived of. If this is correct, then no matter which of the three broad theories about well-being we hold onto (hedonism, desire satisfactionism, or objective list views), it is defensible to claim that there is no distinctive sense in which death is less bad for nonhuman animals – or, in general, for individuals lacking complex cognitive capacities.

Now, two final remarks are in order. First, the previous line of reasoning still holds even if it turns out to be true that most wild animals have unpleasant lives and are not therefore being deprived of a good future by dying. The fact that many wild animals may not be contingently deprived of a good future given the likely prevalence of suffering in their lives does not entail that death may not in principle harm them as much as it would harm a human being with a similar expected level of well-being. In addition, the fact that *some* wild animals may plausibly have lives worth living (e.g., elephants, primates, cetaceans) entails that these animals are, in fact, being deprived of a good future when they die.

Second, recent research in animal cognition has cast serious doubts on the traditional way of thinking about nonhuman animals and death. In particular, the alleged inability of nonhuman animals to have a concept of death would prevent the formation of the relevant desire and thus the possession of the interest in living. It has been suggested that possession of a concept of death, far from being a uniquely human feature, is a fairly common trait in other animals, ranging from chimpanzees to opossums.[27] While it is true that there is much more to learn about animals' understanding of death, at the very least, desire-based views need to be revised so as to accommodate the implications of the possibility of the concept of death requiring much less cognitive complexity, and likely to be widespread among nonhuman animals.[28]

c) Time-Relative Interests

Let us now consider a different account of the harm of death that also differs from the Deprivation Account – the Time-Relative Interest Account, whose first and main proponent is Jeff McMahan.[29] According to the

---

[27] Monsó and Osuna-Mascaró (2020). [28] Monsó (2019). [29] McMahan (2002).

Time-Relative Interest Account, the Deprivation Account of the Badness of Death tells us only part of the truth regarding why death is a harm. It must be further refined in order to accommodate the notion that we can be connected to different degrees with our own future – which in turn conditions the way in which being deprived of it may harm us. On this view, the badness of death is a function of two variables:

(i)   The amount of good P is deprived of at a certain time t_1, considering the value a certain event would have for them at a later time t_2.
(ii) The prudential connection between P at t_1 and P at t_2.

McMahan believes that the prudential connection an individual has with their own future self is determined by the degree to which they are psychologically related to that future. Specifically, in McMahan's words,

> The following relations are instances of *direct psychological connections:* the relation between an experience and a memory of it, the relation between the formation of a desire and the experience of the satisfaction or frustration of that desire, and the relation between an earlier and a later manifestation of a belief, value, intention, or character trait. When there are direct psychological connections between a person P1 at time t1 and a person P2 at t2, P1 and P2 are *psychologically connected* with one another. Because the number of such connections may be many or few, psychological connectedness over time is a matter of degree. It may be strong or weak.[30]

This implies that the interest of P at t_1 in continuing to live is relative to the amount of good P at t_1 loses by dying, discounted by the psychological distance with their future. The least psychologically related the individual is with their future, the less prudentially connected P at t_1 is with their future self (P at t_2), and hence the less P at t_1 is harmed now by not living in the future. In other words, P at t_1's interest in continuing to live weakens in direct proportion to the psychological connection P at t_1 has now with P at t_2.

On the version of the Time-Relative Interest Account defended by McMahan, the case previously discussed regarding the prudential value of Nico's life would now have to be assessed in the other terms. In order to decide whether Nico's death is bad for them, their actual level of well-being must be compared to the well-being they would have had if they remained alive, but now discounted by the degree of psychological connectedness between Nico at t_1 and Nico at t_2. Again, let us assume hedonism and suppose that Nico died at age 20. The total sum of positive and negative experiences Nico suffered during their lifetime results in a net positive amount of 250 units of well-being. Had they remained alive, they would have had 20 more good years and then suffered during their final 5 ones. Had they not died, their lifetime well-being would have been 450. Subtracting this value from their actual lifetime well-being level of 250 gives us − 200. So as to factor in Nico's prudential connection with their future, McMahan suggests we proceed as follows:

> The prudential unity relations in effect function as a multiplier with respect to the value of the event. If, for example, the prudential unity relations would be of maximum strength, we calculate the importance of the event from one's present point of view by multiplying the value the event will have when it occurs by 1; thus the extent to which one ought rationally to be egoistically concerned about the event is proportional to the value the event will contribute to one's life. If, however, the prudential unity relations would be weaker, the extent to which the event matters from one's present point of view declines. We should multiply the value that the event will have when it occurs by some fraction representing the strength of the prudential unity relations. There is, in short, a discount rate for weakened prudential unity.[31]

Then, the disvalue of Nico's dying at 20 must now be calculated by factoring in the degree to which prudential unity relations (i.e., psychological connectedness) would hold between Nico now and Nico at a later time when future valuable events would occur. If their prudential unity relations are of maximum strength, we multiply −200 by 1. The disvalue of Nico's death then coincides on this account with −200. If contrariwise Nico's prudential unity relations are weak (e.g., we can assume that Nico* has a severe mental condition that weakens their prudential unity relations to half the strength of Nico's), then we have to apply a 0.5 fraction to −200. The result then becomes −100. The important implication is that although Nico and Nico* have the same lifetime well-being, the badness of their deaths differs. While Nico is greatly harmed by dying at 20 and thus has a strong interest in continuing to live, Nico* is harmed to a much lesser extent and thus their interest in continuing to live is significantly weaker.

Applied to nonhuman animals, the argument is straightforward. Although death may often deprive nonhuman animals of a life of net positive value, their death cannot be understood as a great misfortune. At least, death is not as bad for them as it is for adult human beings. The reason is that nonhuman animals are usually weakly psychologically

---

[31] Ibid., p. 80.

related to their futures. Due to this psychological discontinuity, when they die, they are deprived of very little and death does not harm them significantly. Thus, a greater discount should be applied when calculating how much nonhuman animals lose in dying. Of course, due to the difference in psychological capacities among nonhuman animals, the discount rate will vary greatly among individuals.

Notwithstanding the prominence of this view, neither the Time-Relative Interest Account nor the way McMahan understands it are immune to criticism. The ways in which it can be disputed have different implications regarding the assessment of the badness of death for nonhuman animals. In any case, the claim that it is worse for humans to die is consistent with the claim that it is extremely bad for nonhuman animals to die, and this could suffice for present purposes. One may, however, challenge McMahan's view.

It is possible to accept the Time-Relative Interest Account, in general, but to reject, in particular, the calculus of the degree of psychological connectedness it assumes. According to Jeff McMahan, an individual's degree of psychological connectedness is directly related to the degree of psychological complexity it possesses. More psychological complexity amounts, according to McMahan, to a greater number of contents of consciousness. As he says,

> An infant is unaware of itself, unaware that it has a future; it therefore has no future directed mental states: no desires or intentions for its future. Because its mental life is so limited, there would be very few continuities of character or belief between itself now and itself as a person. And if it had lived to become a person, it would then remember nothing of its life as an infant. It is, in short, almost completely severed psychologically from itself as it would have been in the future. This is the principal reason why its time-relative interest in continuing to live is so weak. It is almost as if the future it loses might just as well have belonged to someone else.[32]

Hence, an individual with higher cognitive complexity has more contents of consciousness that connect them to their future. Under this assumption, nonhuman animals, who generally possess less complex cognitive capacities, have less contents of consciousness relating them to their future. Therefore, death is not as bad for them as for other individuals with higher cognitive complexity but with a similarly valuable future.

There is, however, some discrepancy regarding the calculation of the degree of psychological connectedness between an individual at some time

---

[32] Ibid., p. 170.

and their future self. For example, it has been claimed that higher complexity (and hence quantity) of mental contents does not necessarily amount to higher psychological connectedness.[33] It is, in fact, possible that an individual with fewer mental contents has higher psychological connectedness than an individual with a higher amount but a more changeable psychology. Consider two individuals with different levels of mental complexity at different points in their existence, as well as their corresponding mental states. This could be represented as follows:

Phoenix:

t_1: {m1, m2, m3, m4, m5, m6, m7, m8}

t_2: {m1, m2, m3, m4, m11, m13, m19, m21}

Quinn:

t_1: {m1, m2, m3, m4}

t_2: {m1, m2, m3, m7}

The first observation is that, compared with Quinn, Phoenix has a greater amount of mental contents that relate them to their future. Thus, according to the Time-Relative Interest Account, Phoenix is more psychologically connected to their future than Quinn and hence their interest in continuing to live is stronger than Quinn's. Nevertheless, though Phoenix's total amount of connected mental contents is greater than the total amount of Quentin's in absolute terms, that is not the case in relative terms. That is, while Phoenix retains 50 percent of their mental contents between t_1 and t_2, Quinn retains 75 percent of them with their future self. One might plausibly claim that what is relevant in determining the degree of psychological connectedness is precisely how much qualitative similarity there is between individuals at some time in their existence and their future selves, and not how many connected mental contents they have in total.

A different example may more clearly illustrate the point. Consider Zoe at a certain time in their life t_1 with a certain amount of mental contents. Imagine two different possible scenarios. At t_2 Zoe has the same amount of mental contents except for one that was irreversibly lost and a new one that appeared. At t_2,' Zoe has been greatly enhanced, such that although all the mental contents they had at t_1 remain at t_2,', at t_2,' they have a huge amount of new mental contents. This could be represented as follows:

---

[33] See Horta (2010c).

Zoe:

t_1 : {m1, m2, m3, m4, m5, m6, m7, m8, m9, m10}

t_2 : {m1, m2, m3, m4, m5, m6, m7, m8, m9, m11}

t_2': {m1, m2, m3, m4, m5, m6, m7, m8, m9, m10, m12, m13, m14, m15, m16, m17, m18, m19, m20, m21, m22, m23, m24, m25, m26, ... m99, m100}

Although Zoe at t_1 is 90 percent connected to Zoe at t_2 and only 10 percent connected to Zoe at t_2', McMahan's account of the Time-Relative Interest Account tells us that the psychological connectedness between Zoe at t_1 and Zoe at t_2' is higher because the total amount of connected mental contents is also higher. But this seems hard to accept. The extent to which this appears to be implausible might be further observed if we conduct a backward-looking assessment of the mental connectedness of Zoe – that is, for instance, between each of Zoe's two possible future scenarios and Zoe at t_1. It then becomes clear that Zoe at t_2' is only very weakly related to their past (i.e., with Zoe at t_1) – only 10 percent connected – whereas Zoe at t_2 is very strongly related to their past (i.e., with Zoe at t_1) – 90 percent connected.

If this proportional approach to the calculus of psychological connectedness is sound, then an individual with less complex psychology does not necessarily have a weaker interest in continuing to live. And if so, nonhuman animals could be as strongly psychologically related to their future (or even more) as the more cognitively endowed individuals (many human beings).

If this is so, then the notion that humans typically lose much more by dying than nonhuman animals, based not only on the assumption that their lives will be better but also because they are more prudentially connected to their own future, can be rejected. This is because although humans may have more mental contents, such mental contents typically vary more throughout their lives. It seems reasonable to think that the mental contents of, say, a mouse will remain more similar throughout their whole life than those of a human being. If this is correct, then the interest in living of human beings and of other animals will not differ in the way that McMahan's version of the Time-Relative Interest Account entails.

Another way to dispute the conclusion that the interest in living of nonhuman animals is comparatively weaker than that of human beings is to endorse a Time-Neutral Account of the badness of death instead. According to such an account, the badness of death is a function of the amount of goods that someone is deprived of at a certain time, which are those that would have accrued to them in the future if they had remained alive. Thus, an individual's interest in being alive depends solely on the full amount of benefits they would have obtained in the future, independently of the psychological distance between the actual individual and their future self. This means that no discount is applied on the basis of diminishing degrees of psychological connectedness.

The major implication of this is that if Phoenix and Quinn have a future of similar net value, then their deaths are similarly bad for them. Hence, their interests in continuing to live are similarly strong, independently of their species or their degree of psychological complexity.

If this is the view we ought to endorse, then the interest in living of human beings and of other animals will depend exclusively on the amount of good (and bad) each of them is deprived of by death. It would not differ in the way the Time-Relative Interest Account entails, either on McMahan's version of it or on the proportional version presented above.

d) *Impersonal Views*

In the previous section, I examined different positions on how to assess the interest in living of nonhuman animals. There remains the alternative, however, of approaching the problem of the badness of death by denying the assumption on which all the previous positions rely. Namely, what has normative importance is the prudential disvalue of death, that is, how bad it is for the individual that ceases to exist. In other words, one can deny that what gives us our reasons against killing, or preventing someone from dying, is the person-affecting value of death. Instead, one might claim that what provides us with such reasons is the badness of death impersonally conceived. If that is the case, then the only thing that matters is the loss of value in the world impartially considered and not to whom that value accrues. For those assuming this view, all other considerations are irrelevant, such as individual desires to continue to live or an individual's relation with their future.

Thus, even if ceasing to exist could not be said to be bad for the one who dies, we would still have reasons to prevent an individual with a life worth living from dying based on the loss of the impersonal value that a life of positive net value would entail. Because the possession of certain desires or of psychological complexity is no longer significant for the badness of death conceived in this way, it follows that the deaths of a nonhuman or a human with a similar future of net positive value are similarly bad. Thus, our reasons to ensure that they continue to exist would be as strong.[34]

On an impersonal view of the badness of death, the fact that humans or other animals die is bad if they would otherwise have had net positive lives. Nonetheless, on this view, their death would not qualify as bad if because of their death other individuals came into existence who had lives of greater net positive value than the first ones would have had. In addition, this view implies that the deaths of humans or other animals would not be bad if their lives had been net negative.

e) Final Remarks

In this section, I examined the problem of the badness of death as applied to nonhuman animals. That is, the problem of whether ceasing to exist may harm animals and, if so, the extent to which it may comparatively harm them relative to human beings. In other words, I assessed the strength of nonhuman interests in continuing to live. I disputed the widespread view according to which, under almost any theoretical assumptions, nonhuman animals lack an interest in being alive or, at most, that the strength of such interest is always comparatively weaker than that of human beings.[35] Given the divergence of competing views on this debate, my conclusions are conditional. If death harms human beings for such and such reasons, then, under the same assumptions, there are many nonhuman animals that are also harmed by ceasing to exist. This allows, of course, for the possibility that often the interest of a human being in continuing to live may be stronger than the interest of a nonhuman animal. Nevertheless, it also allows for the possibility that many times the opposite is the case. Animals can, *in principle*, be as harmed by death as

[34] Singer now explicitly endorses an impersonal view on the badness of death (2015). For a detailed analysis of Singer's commitment to this view, see Paez (2017).

[35] Note that, even so, we could certainly think of many cases in which a nonhuman animal's future has the same surplus of positive value than the future of a human being. Alternatively, we can also think of other cases in which some human beings have a much lower psychological connectedness than some nonhuman individuals. This is the case of human babies and infants, but also of severely cognitively impaired adult human beings. On McMahan's account, because of the greater discount rate that we must apply to these humans' future with lower psychological connectedness, these humans have a weaker interest in continuing to live, and so death is less harmful for them than would be for nonhuman individuals with higher psychological connectedness. Thus, according to this position, the interest in continuing to live of a great number of nonhuman individuals will be stronger than the interest in continuing to live of many human beings. This shows that the interest in continuing to live is not something coextensive to the species individuals belong to but rather variable across and within species.

human beings even if, *in practice*, that might not be common. Therefore, when discussing the badness of death, we must reject the view that human and nonhuman animals harbor fundamental different interests in being alive and favor instead the view that such interest (if it exists) simply varies among individuals across species.

In this chapter, I defended the view that due to their capacity for conscious experiences, nonhuman animals have a well-being of their own – a necessary and sufficient condition to be morally considerable. I further claimed that this is the case independently of the theory of well-being one might endorse (hedonism, the desire-based view, or the objective-list theory). I then argued for the quite uncontroversial claim that nonhuman interests in not suffering are morally relevant and that equal instances of suffering should be equally considered, irrespective of the species individuals belong to. It follows that our reasons to prevent or alleviate nonhuman suffering are as strong as our reasons to prevent equal instances of human suffering.

I then argued for a conditional claim: If death is bad at all, then under certain theoretical assumptions, death is also bad for nonhuman animals and, sometimes, it may be comparatively worse than for human beings. If so, under certain views, the nonhuman interest in continuing to live gives us additional reasons to prevent them from dying. On that assumption, we would thus have not only compelling reasons to prevent or reduce the suffering nonhuman animals endure in the wild but also to avoid their deaths whenever we can – with the proviso that they would have lives of positive net value.

CHAPTER 2

Speciesism

In Chapter 1, I claimed that nonhuman animals are morally considerable and that there are no grounds for considering them disadvantageously in comparison to human beings. This conclusion may nonetheless be disputed if we accept certain views such as speciesism or personism. In this chapter, I assess the cogency of such views and find them wanting.

2.1 The Concept of Speciesism

Despite the increasing attention being recently paid to the different problems in animal ethics, the concept of speciesism remains strikingly overlooked[1]. But what are we exactly talking about when we talk about speciesism? Is it a conceptual truth that speciesism is wrong, or is it a substantive moral judgment? Furthermore, what, if anything, makes speciesism an unjustified position (when it is)? What is the relationship between speciesism and anthropocentrism? These are some contentious issues, and I will not attempt to resolve every one of them here. However, I think it is important to clarify the conceptual dispute by introducing new considerations that will, hopefully, guide us into a more fruitful discussion on this topic.

So, what is speciesism? As a reasonable first approximation, one might say that speciesism is species-based discrimination so that X discriminates Y on the basis of species if, and only if,

(i) There is a property P such that (X believes that) Y has P and (X believes that) Z does not have P.
(ii) X treats Y worse than Z.
(iii) It is because (X believes that) Y has P and Z does not have P that X treats Y worse than Z.

---

[1] Some recent exceptions can be found in Horta and Albersmeir (2020) and Jacquet (2019).

(iv)   P is the property of being a member of a certain species.

Now, on some views, we should add another condition, such that

(v)   The relative disadvantage is unjustified.

Or, we should modify (ii) as follows:

(ii)*   X treats Y unjustifiably worse than Z.

Those who subscribe (v) or (ii)* – commonly called the moralized or evaluative view – believe that speciesism is necessarily wrong. That is, an unjustified instance of relative disadvantage on the basis of species is speciesist, while a justified instance of relative disadvantage on the basis of species simply does not qualify as speciesism. Thus, the sentence "Speciesism is wrong" is a tautology.

The moralized view has been subjected to several criticisms. First, it only allows for a limited usage of the term, and it is inconsistent with some experts' pattern of usage. Second, and most importantly, it seems incompatible with being against or in favor of speciesism, thereby making the philosophical debate on "Is species-based discrimination justified?" unintelligible[2]. Surely, proponents of the view do not see these as fatal criticisms. We need a concept that allows us to condemn certain practices regarding the consideration and treatment of nonhuman animals and a moralized concept allows us to do just that. In order to condemn a certain practice X, we show that X is speciesist. Is X justified? No. X is not justified because X is an instance of speciesism. Potential disagreement then comes down to whether X is an instance of speciesism or not.

Now, those who do not subscribe (v) or (ii)* remain unconvinced. On this other view – commonly called the nonmoralized or descriptive view – "Speciesism is wrong" is not a conceptual truth but rather a substantive moral judgment. In order to condemn a certain practice X, we have to show that X is speciesist *and* that it is wrong (or unjustified). Is X justified? No. X is not justified because it is an unjustified instance of speciesism. Potential disagreement is now on whether X is justified or not.

Surely, the view is also not immune to criticism. First, it overapplies by being unable to distinguish between justified and unjustified differential treatment on the basis of species. Second, it is also inconsistent with some experts' usage of the term, and most importantly it is inconsistent with the colloquial and grass-roots derogatory usage. If we were to adopt it,

[2] Jacquet (2019).

"antispeciesism" would make no sense. Relatedly, it is incompatible with the widespread moralized-evaluative use of analogous terms such as "racism" and "sexism."[3] Of course, the latter might be explained because of the implicature that such instances of discrimination are necessarily unjustified as a matter of moral truth. That is simply omitted in conversation and comes to light when the speaker is prompted to give reasons for their views. At any rate, this would only account for a subset of cases since plausibly not all proponents of a nonmoralized view of "racism" and "sexism" are committed to their being unjustified as a matter of a necessary moral truth.

a)   Ameliorating Speciesism

Now, the debate over the concept of speciesism clearly mimics the debate over the concept of discrimination: Sometimes "speciesism" carries a negative evaluation and other times it is neutral. One way to tackle this problem is to reject the idea that some users and some experts are necessarily misusing the term and instead notice that "speciesism" may simply not be univocal. The following distinction may help us to elucidate this point:

> [w]ith a bit of linguistic ingenuity we can express the distinction we need by separating P-based discrimination, e.g. age-, race- or sex-based discrimination, which involves treating individuals differently depending on their P-properties, but is not necessarily morally objectionable; and P-ist discrimination, e.g. ageist, racist or sexist discrimination, which involves treating individuals differently on the basis of their P-properties in a morally objectionable way. This terminology allows us to say, for example, that proponents of affirmative action for women aim to correct sexist discrimination through sex-based discrimination.[4]

Accordingly, we might arrive at the following distinction:
Species-based discrimination[5]:

(i)   There is a property P such that (X believes that) Y has P and (X believes that) Z does not have P.

---

[3] Horta and Albersmeir 2020; Albersmeir 2021.   [4] Lippert-Rasmussen (2006, pp. 167–168).
[5] The plausibility of the distinction will of course greatly depend on whether we take "discrimination" itself in a moralized or non- moralized sense. If moralized, then "species-based discrimination" should be reformulated into "species-based disadvantageous treatment." Alternatively, some have argued, we could introduce a contrasting, descriptive term in the discussion such as "speciescentrism" (Albersmeier 2021).

(ii)   X treats Y worse than Z.
(iii) It is because (X believes that) Y has P and Z does not have P that X treats Y worse than Z.
(iv)   P is the property of being a member of a certain species.

Speciesist discrimination:

(i)   There is a property P such that (X believes that) Y has P and (X believes that) Z does not have P.
(ii)   X treats Y unjustifiably worse than Z.
(iii) It is because (X believes that) Y has P and Z does not have P that X treats Y worse than Z.
(iv)   P is the property of being a member of a certain species.

The distinction allows us to say that while species-based discrimination is not wrong (or unjustified) by definition, speciesist discrimination is. That allows us to make the philosophical and public debate on whether species-based discrimination is justified intelligible while keeping the derogatory meaning of "speciesism" intact in a way consistent with the evaluative use of analogous terms such as "racism" or "sexism."

There are, of course, other options available. For instance, one might deny that racism or sexism are also wrong by definition. They are both purely descriptive terms, as presumably shown by self-described racists' utterance of sentences like "I am a racist, so what?"[6] I will not engage with this view here, mostly because I fail to see either its theoretical or its sociopolitical advantages. But this particular claim might be dismissed by accepting that while in such sentences the speaker is making a descriptive usage of the term, this could be ruled out as sheer linguistic incompetence. Indeed, the phenomenon seems best captured by a different concept – what Kwame Anthony Appiah called "racialism" – roughly, the belief that there is a biological division between races without implying morally relevant differences between them. According to this view, and along the lines of my previous distinction, some forms of race-based discrimination (or race-based disadvantageous treatment) may be, in principle, justified. "Racism" should instead be reserved for the unjustified race-based forms of discrimination.

Surely, this does not settle which concept of speciesism is preferable. That will depend, in my view, not on the extent to which the proposed definition matches people's intuitions about particular cases (they all fail to

---

[6] Jaquet (2019, p. 454).

a great extent at doing that), but rather on the purposes of our inquiry. In other words, I propose that a good way to think about "speciesism" is by carrying out an ameliorative inquiry[7] into the concept such that instead of aiming "to reveal the operative concept, that is, the objective type that our usage of a certain term tracks (if any)" we aim "to reveal the target concept, that is, the concept that we should be using, given our purposes and goals in [this] inquiry."[8] This way, we will arrive at the concept of speciesism that we should aim to be used, given a particular set of goals.

Notice that proponents of both descriptive and evaluative views not only explore how we currently understand the concept of speciesism but also lay out several reasons for how we should understand it – based on its usefulness. Yet, it still remains unclear for what purposes exactly the concepts are useful. Let's say that our main purpose with the present inquiry is to counteract (wrongful or unjustified) species discrimination, whenever it happens, wherever it happens. Accordingly, the goal of this inquiry is not to think about "speciesism" but rather to engage in antispeciesist theory and show that failing to prevent and reduce the harms that wild animals suffer qualifies as an instance of (wrongful or unjustified) species discrimination – or speciesist discrimination, for short. Therefore, by being in line with one important pattern of theoretical usage as well as by keeping with grass-roots activism, I believe that an evaluative concept will serve the general purpose best.

This section will now examine the relevant elements of the definition separately.

(i) Worse For

The first element of speciesism is that it involves not only differential but also disadvantageous treatment. That is, an agent X treats an individual or group of individuals Y in a way that they do not treat other individuals or group Z in a way that is worse for that individual or group. This entails X inflicting some harm on Y while not inflicting harm on Z at all or only to a lesser extent. Paradigmatic instances of such relative disadvantage include human beings using nonhuman animals for food, clothing, and entertainment while not subjecting members of the human species to the same treatment. Conversely, it entails X failing to provide Y with some benefit or to a lesser extent than to Z. A paradigmatic example of this relative disadvantage includes human beings providing medical care to

---

[7] On the distinction between ameliorative and descriptive inquiries, see the groundbreaking work of Haslanger (2000, 2006). See also Diaz-Leon (2020).
[8] Diaz-Leon (2020, p. 170).

members of the human species while failing to provide medical care to nonhuman animals in similar circumstances.

(ii) Because Of
The second element of speciesism is that agent X treats an individual or group of individuals Y disadvantageously as compared to individuals or group Z *because* X believes individual or group of individuals Z exhibit the property P of belonging to a certain species while individuals or group Y does not. That is, the motivation in support of the disadvantageous consideration or treatment is related to the (perceived) species of individuals. Thus, the disadvantageous consideration or treatment of Y relative to Z is based on the assumption that members of Species 1 possess certain attributes or properties which members of Species 2 do not.

There are three main kinds of such attributes, not to be conceived as mutually exclusive, which have been traditionally advanced in the literature. We may collectively call them *species-specific* attributes:

(a) Mere species membership: Z's membership in S1, which Y fails to possess by being a member of S2. This may assume the biological inferiority of S2 to S1.
(b) Species-specific capacities: the capacities possessed by members of S1, which members of S2 allegedly lack, in virtue of their membership, respectively, in S1 and S2.
(c) Species-specific relations: the relations that Z enters into and Y does not, in virtue of their membership, respectively, in S1 and S2.

The favoring of Z over Y is based, in the first case, on the fact that Z belongs to a certain species and Y does not – thus, on species membership *stricto sensu*. A more sophisticated way to ground this disadvantageous consideration is to base it on certain properties presumably coextensive to the species whose members are being favored. These properties can either be intrinsic to the members of the species (individual capacities) or extrinsic (relations with moral agents). These properties usually work as proxies for species membership.

(iii) In an Unjustifiable Way
The combination of conditions (i) and (ii) is still not sufficient for a position to be speciesist. This is because it may be true that, first, the species-specific attribute is indeed exemplified by all members of S1 and by no member of S2, and that, second, it is a morally relevant attribute justifying the disadvantageous consideration or treatment of members of

S1 over the members of S2. That is, the disadvantageous consideration of an individual based on species membership (broadly understood as to include the three disjuncts (a) to (c) previously mentioned) may be justified. For example, it is usually assumed that while we should assist human beings suffering from natural catastrophes, we have no such obligation to assist nonhuman animals in the exact same circumstances. This difference, it is often argued, can be justified by appeal to certain kinds of special relationships human beings maintain with each other by virtue of belonging to the human community, and which are not maintained with nonhuman animals.[9] If these were morally relevant properties, then we would have reasons in support of certain types of disadvantageous consideration and treatment of nonhuman animals, without thereby incurring in speciesism.

(iii)   A certain position is unjustified, either because the attribute appealed to
        a.   is not species-specific, whether because some Z lack it and/or some Y exhibit it (species overlap test);
             and/or
        b.   is irrelevant for the moral consideration or treatment of individuals (relevance test).

Whenever the attribute in question is not species-specific, that is, whenever there are members of both S1 and of S2 who lack them or who possess them, we can say that there is a *species overlap*. Therefore, one way in which a position may be unjustified is if there is a species overlap regarding the attribute invoked to ground the differential consideration. For instance, consider the individual capacity of *moral agency*. There is a species overlap if at least one member of S2 that qualifies as a moral agent or at least one member of S1 that does not qualify as such. Now consider the relation of *solidarity*. There is a species overlap if at least one member of S2 enters into a relation of solidarity with moral agents or at least one member of S1 does not enter into any such relation.[10]

Another way in which a certain position may be unjustified is if the allegedly species-specific attribute invoked to establish the disadvantageous consideration among individuals is not relevant for how they ought to be

---

[9] Palmer (2010).
[10] For a detailed analysis of the argument from species overlap (sometimes also called the argument from marginal cases), see Horta (2014). See also Singer (1975); Dombrowski (1996; 2006); Pluhar (1995); Ehnert (2002); Bernstein (2002); Norcross (2004); Wilson (2005), Tanner (2011a).

considered. This is not an empirical matter, and it requires a further argument. Nevertheless, it allows us to dismiss those attempts to ground instances of disadvantageous consideration or treatment in actual (or alleged) biological differences between Y and Z that are unimportant to how the individual interests at stake will be affected. Consider, for example, the claim that, in similar circumstances, it is justified to inflict a certain amount of pain on a nonhuman animal, but not on a human being, because human beings are moral agents. This claim assumes that possession of moral agency is relevant to how individual interests are to be taken into account. As I will later discuss in this chapter, however, this can be disputed. If possession of moral agency is irrelevant for moral consideration, then this would be an unjustified position.

We can arrive, thus, at the following definition of speciesism:

> *Speciesism (Wide Definition):* the unjustified disadvantageous consideration or treatment of an individual x over another y, either by appeal to their species membership or by appeal to other allegedly species-specific attributes that members of x's species are believed to lack and that members of y's species are believed to possess.

b)   The Overspeciesism Objection

It might be objected that under such a definition we are allowed to classify as speciesist positions that ground the disadvantageous consideration or treatment of some individuals not directly on their species but on their lack of certain species-specific capacities and relations. These would be positions not normally classified as such. I will call this the *Overspeciesism Objection*. The claim is not that there might be a view that is "extremely speciesist" or "too speciesist,"[11] but that the definition presented above is overinclusive: It calls speciesist views that are not strictly speciesist. In this section, I will thus refer to the definition defended here as the *Wide Definition* of speciesism, as opposed to the definition that prevails in the literature. The question at stake here, therefore, is whether the *Wide Definition* is too wide, so much so that it is not an adequate one.

Now in order to determine what is the prevalent definition in the literature, let us first consider the "Declaration against Speciesism" proclaimed at Cambridge in 1977. There it is said that "We do not accept that a difference in species alone (any more than a difference in race) can justify

---

[11] Further below, I will argue against the claim that a view can be "extremely speciesist."

wanton exploitation or oppression."[12] Indeed it seems clear that the authors were using "speciesism" to denote a narrower kind of unjustified disadvantageous consideration. Thus,

> *Speciesism (Narrow Definition)*: Speciesism is the unjustified disadvantageous consideration or treatment of an individual x over another y by appeal to their species membership alone.

Several authors in the literature[13] endorse the *Narrow Definition*. They consider that if a position allows for the disadvantageous consideration of members of a certain species by appeal to individual capacities or relations they allegedly possess, which are considered morally relevant, it is not a speciesist position (although it may be unjustified for other reasons). The implication would be then that these other types of unjustified disadvantageous consideration or treatment of individuals who do not belong to a certain species ought not to be classified as speciesist, but differently.

Nevertheless, it is worth asking what further reasons we may have to prefer the *Narrow* over the *Wide Definition* of speciesism. There seems to be a common worry that, if we take "speciesism" too broadly, that will lead us to label some famous animal ethicists such as Peter Singer as speciesist as well. That would somehow be a sign that something must be wrong with our definition and that it should thus be revised. Rojer Fjellstrom seems to have this in mind when he writes,

> Are there any philosophical opinions favoring humans that do not invoke typical human properties? Also, Singer and Rachels would become unqualified speciesists in this way, since they defend the higher value of human life by pointing to the typical human property of having a biographical life.[14]

The implication is that, since that would be absurd, we should reject that way of understanding speciesism. Thus, classifying Singer's position as speciesist would somehow be a *reductio* of speciesism so defined.

However, it seems that the definition of speciesism should not be appraised by such contingent facts, such as whether Singer's position could be classified as speciesist or not.[15] The mere fact that one names a prejudice (or, in this case, popularizes it) does not make one immune to it. So, unless we are willing to oppose the definition on an argument from authority, such considerations are not pertinent to this discussion. To be sure, I'm not endorsing the claim that Peter Singer is speciesist. Indeed,

---

[12] See Paterson and Ryder (1979).   [13] Salient examples include Ryder (1970); Singer (1975).
[14] Fjellstrom (2002, p. 69).
[15] For the speciesist charge on Singer (and the Great Ape Project), see Sapontzis (1993, pp. 269–277).

under the definition I am advancing, this could hardly be claimed. The point is that even if that followed, from my view, it would not be a reason against it.

The Overspeciesism Objection does not succeed, ultimately, because by adopting a *Narrow Definition* of speciesism we would be excluding from that category relevant instances of unjustified discrimination based on the species to which individuals belong.

One way in which this can be observed is by considering the following. "Racism" is usually taken as unjustified disadvantageous consideration of those who do not have certain physical traits socially recognized as related to ethnicity or race. "Sexism," on its part, is usually employed as the unjustified disadvantageous consideration of those who are not classified as belonging to a certain sex. If we were to accept as narrow a conception of racism and sexism as the one considered here for speciesism, only those positions strictly based on membership in a certain race or sex *alone* could be classified as racist or sexist. On the contrary, a position that entailed the disadvantageous consideration of certain individuals on account of their putatively inferior cognitive capacities, which they are supposed to possess in virtue of their race or sex, could not be classified as racist or sexist. However unjustified these positions might be, it would not follow that they were racist or sexist, technically speaking. However, it seems that there is an important sense in which they are. Or, more to our point, an important sense in which they *should* be. Using a certain proxy for excluding individuals who are perceived as belonging to a certain sex or race should also qualify as unjustified sex- or race-based forms of discrimination. Such phenomena have profoundly devastating effects on individuals by making (or are reasonably expected to make) perceived members of certain groups worse off than the rest of the population. If our aim is to correct for race- and wrongful discrimination, we need wide concepts of racism and sexism to target these "peculiar" disadvantages imposed on such individuals. Likewise, we need a wide concept of speciesism to encompass all the disadvantages imposed on nonhumans.

These concepts coincide in their structure. If we insist that "racism" and "sexism" should apply to all those instances of disadvantageous consideration that do not strictly appeal to group membership, then "speciesism" should also be held to apply to those instances of disadvantageous consideration that do not strictly appeal to membership in a species. Rather, we should use these terms to cover instances of unjustified discrimination based on other alleged group-specific attributes, such as individual capacities or relations. Thus, if we rejected the *Wide Definition*, we would necessarily leave relevant instances of species-based unjustified discrimination out. Because we ought not, the Overspeciesism Objection fails.

2.2 Speciesism and Anthropocentrism

"Speciesism" is often used to refer to the unjustified favoring of human beings over members of other species.[16] The unwarranted assumption underlining this usage is that speciesism and anthropocentrism are equivalent terms. Anthropocentrism can be characterized as follows:

> *Anthropocentrism*: Human beings are fully morally considerable, whereas nonhuman animals are either morally considerable to a lesser extent or not considerable at all.

(a) Alleged Equivalence

There are two ways in which the equivalence of speciesism and anthropocentrism may be understood, each of them giving rise to different problems. The first understanding of "speciesism" and "anthropocentrism" as equivalent terms can be observed in several attempts to define speciesism in the literature. While they do not explicitly assert it, they certainly presuppose it. Here are some famous examples:

> I use the word "speciesism" to describe the widespread discrimination that is practiced by man against the other species, and to draw a parallel with racism.[17]

> Speciesism is the inclusion of all human animals within, and the exclusion of all other animals from, the moral circle.[18]

> A speciesist position, at least the paradigm of such a position, would take the form of declaring that no animal is a member of the moral community because no animal belongs to the "right" species – namely, Homo sapiens.[19]

These definitions are problematic since a position is conceivable such that (i) it would prescribe an unjustified preferential consideration of members of a particular nonhuman species against the rest of them. Imagine, for example, that someone maintains that only birds should be given moral consideration and that their interests should always be preferred over the interests of other nonhuman species, the reason being that this person likes

---

[16] Some parts of this section have been discussed in Faria and Paez (2014).   [17] Ryder (1983, p. 5).
[18] Waldau (2001, p. 38).   [19] Regan (1985, p. 155).

birds but does not feel any sympathy for other nonhuman animals. It seems as if this person is being speciesist, insofar as it is favoring the members of a certain species (nonhuman) over the members of another (nonhuman), based on an unjustified appeal to their relation of sympathy toward the members of certain species (birds). They are not being anthropocentric, though, since they are not favoring human interests over nonhuman ones.

In addition, it could also be the case that a certain position (ii) prescribed an unjustified disadvantageous consideration of members of a particular nonhuman species, though not of all of them. Imagine that someone claims that all sentient nonhuman animals should be morally considerable, except rats, whom they find repugnant. It seems that this person is establishing an unjustified differentiation among individuals based on their relation of repugnancy with all the members of a certain species. They are clearly being speciesist, though hardly anthropocentric, since they are not giving preferential consideration or treatment to humans over nonhumans, but rather considering the members of a certain nonhuman species (rats) against the members of other species, in an unjustified disadvantageous way.

b)   *Alleged Inevitability*

There is another way in which the equivalence between anthropocentrism and speciesism might be understood, namely by claiming that anthropocentrism implies speciesism. As before, this claim has not been explicitly endorsed by philosophers, though it is often presupposed in their arguments. This is a very strong claim that gives rise to significant problems beyond the conceptual realm. Usually, the equivalence does not aim at restricting the scope of "speciesism" to the human species, but rather aims at justifying it. The claim may be made more intelligible taken as a premise being part of an argument:

(i)   Because anthropocentrism is inevitable, it is justified.
(ii)   Speciesism is equivalent to anthropocentrism.
(iii) Therefore, speciesism is justified.

This argument requires careful examination due to the ambiguity of the terms being used. It seems that in (i) "anthropocentrism" refers to the fact that human beings are epistemically determined to understand the world anthropocentrically. That is, human beings are such that the limits and form of their knowledge necessarily take the human reference. For instance, human beings understand themselves and make sense of their practices in terms of species identity and partiality toward their fellow humans. Call this *epistemic anthropocentrism*. This being so, humans cannot help but think "humanly," and thus anthropocentrism is justified.

Regarding premise (ii), we have already provided sound reasons to reject it. However, even if we grant it some plausibility, it should be disputed for independent reasons. In (ii), "anthropocentrism" is used with a different meaning, that is, to denote the belief that the satisfaction of human interests has priority over the interests of nonhumans. Call this *moral anthropocentrism*. This is problematic since epistemic anthropocentrism is not equivalent to moral anthropocentrism. While the first is a description about the epistemic equipment of human beings, the second one is a criterion for moral consideration. Most importantly, moral anthropocentrism does not follow from epistemic anthropocentrism. The fact that human beings are endowed in a certain way for their understanding of the world does not imply that they are justified in giving moral priority to the satisfaction of human interests.

Nevertheless, these are precisely the grounds of common arguments against speciesism. The famous philosopher Bernard Williams, for example, writes,

> The word "speciesism" has been used for an attitude some regard as our ultimate prejudice in favor of humanity. It is more revealingly called "humanism," and it is not a prejudice. To see the world from a human point of view is not an absurd thing for human beings to do.[20]

We can now explicitly formulate the argument as follows:

(i) Epistemic anthropocentrism is equivalent and/or implies moral anthropocentrism.
(ii) Epistemic anthropocentrism is justified.
(iii) Therefore, moral anthropocentrism is justified.

Given that

(iv) Moral anthropocentrism is equivalent to speciesism,
(v) Speciesism is justified.

Yet (v) does not follow. For the reasons exposed, (iii) is not the case. In addition, we should reject (iv), since the equivalence between moral anthropocentrism and speciesism is unwarranted.

---

[20] Williams (1985, p. 118; see also 2006).

In conclusion, two important problems arise from a confusion between anthropocentrism and speciesism. The first one follows from an equivalence between moral anthropocentrism and speciesism. This is problematic because many unjustified differentiations of members of nonhuman species would not be classified as speciesist, despite clearly satisfying the requirements. The second one is by claiming that anthropocentrism implies (and justifies) speciesism. This is nevertheless unwarranted. Moral anthropocentrism does not follow from epistemic anthropocentrism and the justification for epistemic anthropocentrism does not justify moral anthropocentrism. Even if speciesism were equivalent to moral anthropocentrism, it would not be justified on the basis that (epistemic) anthropocentrism might be.

c) Alleged Justification

Moral anthropocentrism is incompatible with the principle of equal consideration of interests. In order to assess whether it is, nevertheless, justified, we need to examine whether the arguments provided to defend it succeed. There have been different attempts to defend anthropocentrism. This is typically done by appealing to certain attributes supposedly coextensive with the human species and which would ground the greater moral consideration of its members.[21]

One way to argue for moral anthropocentrism is simply to claim that membership in the human species is morally relevant, that is, by appealing to a definitional defense of anthropocentrism. Yet this seems a clear example of an arbitrary position, as it consists merely in stating that a certain biological classification is morally important. However, there are other attributes that have been defended as supposedly coextensive with membership in the human species. The more prominent candidates include such capacities as autonomy, self-awareness, rationality or speech, and affective, social, or political relations.

---

[21] See Narveson (1977); Frey (1988); Leahy (1991); Carruthers (1992); Scruton (1996) ; or Petrinovich (1999). Though this is the most sophisticated attempt to defend speciesism, it is not the only one that has been employed. On most occasions, moral anthropocentrism is simply asserted as true, rather than argued for, perhaps characterizing it as a basic, nonrevisable moral belief. Since, however, it is possible to give arguments against it and many individuals have abandoned the position, it is indeed revisable. Alternatively, it has sometimes been claimed that moral anthropocentrism is true because humans have souls, or are especially related to a deity. But since we have no evidence that such things are the case, we have no reasons to adhere to moral anthropocentrism on those grounds.

In the past decades, nonetheless, the cogency of these arguments in defense of anthropocentrism has been widely challenged.[22] Consider any of the mentioned attributes (autonomy, self-awareness, rationality or speech, and affective, social, or political relations) that would justify that all nonhuman animals have no moral consideration, or less moral consideration, than all human beings. For any of these attributes to perform the intended justificatory function, it must be the case that the corresponding criterion

(a) is exemplified by all human beings and, at the same time, is not exemplified by any nonhuman being;

and

(b) is morally relevant.

However, none of the aforementioned attributes satisfies these conditions. Let us start with requirement (a). Whatever attribute we may use to draw a moral boundary between humans and nonhumans will either fail to be exemplified by all humans or will be possessed as well by some nonhumans. This is commonly called the phenomenon of *species overlap*.[23] It follows from this phenomenon that for any candidate attribute, one must face a dilemma – either to exclude some human beings from the scope of full moral consideration (e.g., those who lack certain cognitive capacities) or to extend such scope to include also nonhuman animals. Nevertheless, it can hardly be denied that human beings who lack some cognitive capacities or fail to enter into affective, social, or political relations possess full moral consideration. Most of us find that view clearly unacceptable.

One criterion that grants all sentient human beings moral consideration is sentience. But then, this is a criterion that not only they will satisfy, but also any other sentient animals. This means that if we accept a criterion that deprives nonhuman animals of full consideration, that criterion will also exclude a number of sentient human beings. If, instead, we want to agree on a (not merely definitional) moral criterion that will not deprive any sentient human being of moral consideration, that criterion will be one that cannot be used to defend moral anthropocentrism. It is worth noting that even if sentience did not extend to animals, it still wouldn't justify moral anthropocentrism. This is because not all human beings are

---

[22] See, for instance, Dunayer (2004); Horta (2010b); Pluhar (1995); Regan (1983); or Singer (2002).
[23] For a detailed analysis of the scope of this argument, see Horta (2014).

sentient, a paradigmatic example being anencephalic infants. Sentience justifiably excludes some human beings.

This conclusion also seems sound regarding the second criterion – that the attribute appealed to must be relevant for moral consideration. As already explained in Chapter 1, the view that having a well-being is what matters for moral consideration seems to be a very cogent one. It was additionally argued that sentience is a necessary and sufficient condition for an individual to have a well-being of their own. Since sentience is precisely the capacity that makes it possible for a being to be affected in positive (pleasure) and negative ways (suffering), moral consideration should therefore be extended to include all sentient nonhuman beings as well. If we agree on this, then for anthropocentrism to be justified it ought to be grounded in another criterion for moral consideration that is in itself relevant as well for having a well-being.

Certainly, there are many attributes that can be *indirectly* relevant for well-being in certain circumstances. Being able to enjoy coffee or literature, for instance, can be so, as enjoying such things, or being deprived thereof, can increase or reduce our well-being. Yet these attributes cannot pass the "relevance test." That is, for them to be relevant for moral considerability, they would have to be something that *determines* that someone is morally considerable. In the case of the criteria mentioned above (autonomy, self-awareness, rationality or speech, and affective, social, or political relations), we can claim that something similar happens. They can certainly be indirectly relevant for having a well-being. This means that in some cases they will be important to make a moral decision concerning the interests of those who have them. But these attributes are not what determines that someone can have a well-being – only sentience is. If that is so, then we can conclude that all these criteria fail to pass the "relevance test" as well. Therefore, they cannot affect the attribution of full moral considerability.

Some might worry that even if attributes such as autonomy and rationality fail to pass the *species overlap* test, it is still not clear that they fail to pass the "moral relevance test." Consider, for instance, the capacity for reciprocity. It seems that it is relevant to whether a being's interests warrant consideration. If a being can't consider my interests, some might ask, why must I consider theirs? Notice, however, that despite being echoed by a certain common-sense morality, rationality and autonomy are usually not understood as relational properties in the sense that seems to be implied by the objection. According to standard views, the possession of complex cognitive capacities does not require the capacity to relate to others in mutually responsive ways, but merely engaging in certain cognitively complex acts or responses on their own.

To clarify how complex cognitive capacities fail to pass both tests, it is perhaps helpful to introduce the distinction between a property being relevant for the purposes of (i) moral consideration, a property being relevant as a (ii) source of additional moral obligations, and a property being relevant (iii) for the purposes of distinguishing between those individuals who are able to owe moral obligations and those who are unable to owe them.

Accordingly, a property is relevant for (i) only if it determines a being's capacity to receive harms and benefits. While it is reasonable to believe that rationality and autonomy determine the type of harms and benefits a being may receive, it does not determine a being's capacity to receive harms and benefits itself. In that sense, autonomy and rationality are irrelevant for the purposes of *which beings* should be morally considered, while they may remain relevant to *how* those beings should be considered. For instance, they may constitute a source of additional moral obligations and, on occasions, lead to a difference in the strength of reasons for how harms and benefits are allocated among equally morally considerable beings. Likewise, it could be said, certain complex cognitive capacities are necessary for moral agency. Beings who lack those capacities are unable to owe moral obligations although others may owe moral obligations to them.

In light of all this, considering what the argument from *species overlap* and the argument from relevance claim, we can conclude that the criteria presented to defend moral anthropocentrism cannot be considered successful. If those arguments are sound, the implication is that moral anthropocentrism is an unjustified view.

Once we acknowledge that sentience is sufficient for full moral considerability, all other distinctions on which to base the disadvantageous consideration or treatment of the interests of individuals are shown to be arbitrary. Thus, it is unjustified to give greater weight to a particular interest in not suffering of a human being than to a similar interest of a dog. Yet it is likewise unjustified to give greater weight to a particular interest in not suffering of a dog than to a similar interest of a cow. Therefore, not only anthropocentrism but all kinds of non-anthropocentric speciesism must be rejected.

Now, some might accept this conclusion and disagree on the reasons why speciesism is wrong or an unjustified position. For instance, new emphasis has recently been placed on the idea that speciesism is wrong due to species membership being a merely biological property, and merely biological properties are irrelevant to the consideration we owe an entity.[24] Yet, in my view, the wrongness of speciesism need not (and perhaps should not) presuppose that being human (and nonhuman) is a biological property. It is plausible to think that the species category would be better defined in terms of individuals' social position.[25] In that sense, being human (and nonhuman) should be understood in terms of how one is socially perceived, viewed, and treated rather than in terms of biological differences with other species.

It is certainly true that our practices of species categorization do not always track accurate biological classifications. We perceive and treat differently, dogs and dingos, pigs and wild boars, and wild and domestic cats, without those differences corresponding to any biological fruitful distinction. Plausibly, part of the nature of being a pig, a dog, or a cat is to stand in a certain relation to specific social practices. Additionally, the fact that what it means to be a human (and nonhuman) differs across time and place suggests that its conceptual boundaries are contingent on social events and arrangements.

That being said, I am not committing myself to rejecting biological realism about species. Yet, I do believe that our framework for analyzing the justification or wrongness of speciesism should allow us to remain neutral with regard to the nature of species membership.[26] Species membership may be better defined as a social property and still be irrelevant for the purposes of who should be morally considered. In addition, it should also allow that a position using a certain proxy for species membership (e.g., cognitive complexity) with the aim of excluding nonhuman animals from moral consideration might also qualify as (wrongful) speciesism, even if the attribute being used as a proxy is not a merely biological property.

On a different note, some might claim that speciesist views should nevertheless be positioned in a sort of scale of plausibility, depending on how close or farther away they stand from what would count as a proper justification for a disadvantageous consideration. James Rachels, for example, offers one such distinction between *radical speciesism* and *mild speciesism*.[27] He claims that while *radical speciesism* prescribes giving priority to

---

[24] Jaquet (2020).
[25] Cora Diamond (1978, 1991) has defended the claim that being human understood as a social property actually grounds human moral exceptionalism. For convincing criticisms, see McMahan (2005).
[26] Consider the unwelcome implications a similar reasoning would have for the wrongness of sexism depending on sex and race qualifying as merely biological properties.
[27] Rachels (1990).

the satisfaction of trivial human interests over life-sustaining interests of animals (e.g., human gastronomical pleasures override animal suffering in the factory farm), *mild speciesism* prescribes favoring human interests only when comparable nonhuman interests are at stake (e.g., life or death situation or involving the same amount of pain).[28]

However, it is not clear in what way a *mild* speciesist position is, in any relevant sense, closer to being justified than a *radically* speciesist one is. There is a difference between a position being justified and a position being widely accepted. What seems to be the case though is that since *radical* and *mild speciesism* accord different levels of considerability to nonhuman animals, they differ, at least in practice, on the level of acceptance they gain from most people. Most human beings share anti-cruelty intuitions that could not be accommodated by *radical speciesism*: They would not accept the idea that it is justified to satisfy the most trivial human interests over the interests of nonhuman animals in being alive.

Yet a position that prescribes the moral consideration of nonhuman animals in some respects but not in others is no more justified than a position that prescribes a complete disregard of nonhuman interests. Such justification depends solely on the moral relevance of the properties being invoked. If a certain property is not relevant to establish the disadvantageous consideration of certain individuals regarding, for example, their life-sustaining interests, then that property is irrelevant, whether those interests are being disregarded in favor of trivial or life-sustaining human interests.

Rachels also makes a distinction between *qualified* and *unqualified* speciesism. Here Rachels points to a qualitative difference between the arguments used to defend speciesism, according to the strength of the reasons provided. *Unqualified speciesism* refers to those positions that do not advance any arguments in support of the priority of human interests (e.g., definitional defenses). *Qualified speciesism*, on the other hand, goes beyond a mere definitional defense of speciesism and provides reasons in support of favoring the members of some species over the members of another (e.g., appealing to moral agency capacity).

This distinction, however, is also problematic. For it seems to presuppose that *qualified speciesism* is more reasonable than *unqualified speciesism*. Whatever the precise meaning of "reasonable," it should nonetheless not to be confused with "justified." In fact, what seems to be the case is that *qualified speciesism* is merely based on a more complex argument – an

---

[28] Zamir (2007), for instance, would fall under such category in what regards, at least, life or death situations.

appeal to species-specific attributes other than species membership. Yet, as we have seen before, the justification of a moral position solely depends on the resistance of such attributes to *species overlap* and to the relevance test. And *qualified speciesism* does not seem better at resisting these challenges than *unqualified speciesism*. Though its higher complexity allows it not to beg the question, *qualified speciesism* does not resist the argument from species overlap nor the moral relevance test.

Moreover, the distinctions made by Rachels seem inadequate since they give the wrong impression that to be a *mild* or *qualified speciesist* is more justified than being a *radical* or *unqualified* speciesist. However, the lack of justification is the same, as it can be clearly gathered from the following test. Consider the following *qualified, mild speciesist* position:

(a)   The life-sustaining interests of human beings should be favored over the life-sustaining interests of nonhuman beings since human beings, by virtue of belonging to the human species, engage in relations of solidarity with other human beings but do not engage in those relations with nonhuman beings.

Now we may substitute "human beings" by "males" and "nonhuman beings" by "non-males," as follows:

(b)   The life-sustaining interests of males should be favored over the life-sustaining interests of non-males since males, by virtue of belonging to a certain sex/gender, engage in relations of solidarity with other men but do not engage in those relations with non-males.

It is clear how the "reasonability" of the first claim can only be explained by a speciesist bias since both claims are unjustified to the same extent: Both considerations are based on morally irrelevant properties. However, it seems that the lack of justification only becomes apparent once we substitute the category of species for that of sex/gender. And clearly, we would not consider it appropriate to call (b) qualified mild sexism because that would wrongly suggest that such a position would be less sexist (thus, more justified) than a more radical, unreasoned form of it.

However, both versions of sexism, because they are equally unjustified, are equally sexist. They both prescribe an unjustified disadvantageous consideration of those who do not belong to a certain sex/gender, based on a morally irrelevant property (relation of solidarity). And there are no good reasons to think differently in the case of speciesism: What seems to be determinant in identifying a position as speciesist is not the extent to which it excludes some individuals from moral consideration, but only if the criteria used to exclude them are morally relevant.

Speciesism is thus more accurately understood as a categorical notion, not admitting of degrees. Independently of the sophistication of the reasons provided to support a certain disadvantageous consideration and its extent, a certain position cannot be more or less speciesist; either it is or it is not.

This is, of course, compatible with adopting a gradual description of different forms of speciesism, for classificatory and practical purposes more generally. That is, one may say that, at the purely descriptive level, "speciesism" refers to a huge set of views, which range from positions close to antispeciesism, others very far from it, and many somewhere in between. It might be helpful, pragmatically speaking, to rank those positions according to the amount of disvalue they bring or would bring about in a nonideal world. Yet, the classification itself says nothing about the level of justification attached to those views. I leave it as an open question whether such a classification, all things considered, should be used.

2.3 Personism

Some might dispute the relevance of this discussion by saying that most human beings are not actually speciesists. Instead, they are personists, so there is where the discussion should be. This is the path recently followed by Shelly Kagan in an attempt to offer an alternative account of what it is that makes it justifiable to favor the interests of all humans over the like interests of other animals – a view which Kagan calls "modal personism".

There have been many attempts in the literature to justify the claim that persons are morally considerable to a higher extent than nonpersons.[29] It is not the aim of this section to assess general personhood approaches, although the end of the chapter makes some brief remarks on that debate. For the time being, I will leave open the question of their justifiability. Instead, I will focus exclusively on Kagan's view. The reason is that the general aim of this chapter is to dispute the claim that there is some species-specific attribute humans possess that justifies the disadvantageous consideration of nonhuman animals. While Kagan argues for the existence

[29] See McCloskey (1979); Melden (1980); White (1989); Carruthers (1992).

of such an attribute, that need not be true of other versions of personism.[30] Thus,

> *Modal personism*: The interests of individuals who are either (a) *actual* persons or (b) *modal* persons (nonpersons who could have been persons) count more than the like interests of other nonpersons.

This might, in principle, qualify as a speciesist position on this chapter's definition. This is because Kagan considers the property of being a modal person to be a species-specific attribute, and therefore possessed by all members of a species – any species, not necessarily *Homo sapiens* – simply in virtue of being members of that species (of course, in addition, in order to qualify as speciesist it would also have to be morally irrelevant).[31] As Kagan puts it,

> [T]his view does not insist that there is something uniquely special about being a *Homo sapiens* per se, being a member of that *particular* species. But it does hold that species membership can matter morally: so long as you are a member of a species, any species, whose typical adult members are *persons* – call this a "person species" – that suffices to have your interests count more.[32]

This is why Kagan believes that most of us are personists, in this sense, rather than speciesists. We favor the interests of persons (self-conscious individuals) – actual or modal – over the interests of nonperson animals (merely sentient beings).

According to Kagan, as stated, a modal person is a nonperson individual who could have been a person. There is, of course, a way in which any individual P could have been a person, in the sense that there is a possible world in which P's counterpart is a person. Kagan is well aware of this, so he concedes that perhaps modal personhood should be understood as a matter of degree. The possible world in which P's counterpart is a person may be more or less remote from the actual world in which P is a nonperson. He also suggests that there might be a threshold of closeness such that, beyond it, the fact that P is a modal person has moral relevance, whereas below that threshold it does not.[33]

What Kagan suggests, then, is that we should consider that the worlds that are close enough to the actual one for moral purposes are at least those

---

[30] For views that take personhood to be grounded in mere sentience, see Aaltola (2008); Sztybel (2008); and also Faria (2011).
[31] For similar views, see Cohen (1986); see also Cohen and Regan (2001); White (1989); Scruton (1996); Schmidtz (1998).
[32] Kagan (2016), p. 12.   [33] Ibid. p. 19.

in which P's counterparts belong to the same species as P, provided that P's species is what Kagan calls a *person-species*. A person-species is one whose typical adult members are persons. If an individual belongs to a person-species, then that individual could have been a person in the morally relevant way. They are a modal person. Therefore, on this view, the morally relevant property is that of being a modal person – and not species membership per se.[34]

Modal personism is open to several challenges. First, assuming that being a counterfactual person matters, then it seems that being a person in the future ought to matter as well. Indeed, it may matter even more since the latter populates the actual world, but the former does not. Yet Kagan's account of modal personhood excludes *potential persons*,[35] that is, actual nonpersons who will become persons. In line with what has been pointed out by Jeff McMahan, this can lead us to conclude – quite implausibly – that most anencephalic individuals (modal persons) are morally considerable to a greater extent than sentient fetuses and cognitively typical infants (potential, but not modal, persons).[36]

If, instead, Kagan bites the bullet and accepts that potential persons should also be considered for moral purposes his position will run into additional counterintuitive scenarios. Namely, the implication that conscious fetuses are to be considered to a greater extent than cognitively impaired human adults with similar cognitive capacities. This is because while the first actually have the potential to become persons and thus are very close to being one, the second never had such potential and thus are much more distant from being persons. Hence, despite their having similar cognitive capacities, the interests of impaired human adults have less moral weight than the like interests of fetuses.[37]

Second, if closeness to the actual world is what matters to determine the relevance of the modal property at issue, then we may question the way of identifying the relevant closeness of the possible worlds by appealing to species membership. This is something that has been pointed out both by David De Grazia[38] and Jeff McMahan[39] using the following thought experiment. Suppose that at some point it were possible to artificially enhance dogs through genetic modification such that they would

---

[34] For a more detailed analysis and defense of modal personism, see Kagan (2019). A full critique of such view is outside the scope of this chapter. At any rate, it only affects the relative intensity of our obligations to animals, not their existence.

[35] Positions that appeal to the potential personhood of human beings have been extensively challenged in the literature. See, for instance, Pluhar (1995); Nobis (2004); Cavalieri (2001).

[36] Kagan (2016, p. 3).   [37] Ibid., p. 4.   [38] De Grazia (2016).   [39] McMahan (2016).

incrementally become persons in a way that is identity-preserving. If this became possible, then dogs (or other nonperson animals for that matter) ought to be considered modal persons in the relevant way. Moreover, suppose further that turning them into persons were easy and required very little effort. In that case, they would be closer to being a person than a current cognitively impaired human adult is. This, although dogs would still not be members of a person-species. Ultimately what must matter for modal personism is how close the possible world in which the individual is a person is to the actual world. This is not, however, a view that can offer support for the claim that species membership, even if derivatively, can be a relevant criterion.[40]

Finally, we can dispute the general personhood approach (based on actual or modal properties). Indeed, the appeal to personhood as a basis for favoring human interests over nonhumans ones has been under permanent attack in the literature.[41] The debate is dominated by two main positions: (i) the position that disputes that being a person is a species-specific property and (ii) the position that disputes that personhood is a morally relevant property altogether. Regarding (i), even assuming that it were possible to draw a clear line between persons and nonpersons (usually, based on a cluster of complex cognitive capacities), it would still not be possible to avoid *species overlap*. That is, some human individuals would fail to qualify as persons (by lacking some of the specified cognitive capacities) while some nonhumans would definitely qualify as such (by exemplifying some of those capacities).[42] The implication is, then, straightforward: While the interests of the former matter, the interests of the latter do not, or, if they do matter, it is to a much lesser extent.

One might say, however, that this is precisely the point where Kagan's modal personism succeeds where other traditional appeals to personhood fail. This is because, on Kagan's account, those under the *species overlap* would not be excluded from moral considerability since they would either qualify as actual persons (nonhumans who possess the relevant capacities) or as modal persons (humans who do not possess those capacities but could have possessed them in virtue of belonging to a species whose typical members possess the capacities). Yet, and again, the extent to which human nonpersons qualify as modal persons while nonhuman nonpersons

---

[40] For a different approach to critiquing Kagan's view, see Jaquet (2020).
[41] See, for example, Sapontzis (1987); De Grazia (1997); Dunayer (2004); Donaldson and Kymlicka (2011a).
[42] See, for instance, Cavalieri and Singer (1993); White (2007); Poole (1998); Cavalieri (2006).

do not would still be highly questionable on the grounds provided by De Grazia and McMahan. Given the possibility, in principle if not yet in practice, of nonhuman cognitive enhancement, nonhuman animals are as close to being a person as a current cognitively impaired human adult – or even, perhaps, closer. Therefore, they should not be excluded from qualifying as modal persons either.

Alternatively, regarding position (ii), we have reasons to reject the whole personhood framework. Whatever attribute or set of attributes we may appeal to in order to define personhood, it will greatly vary across human beings (as well as across an individual's life). The implication is that the extent to which human interests matter should then be correspondingly adjusted, allowing for the interests of the least endowed human beings to be sacrificed for the benefit of the best endowed.

A personist might respond to this by claiming that personhood (or its underlying capacities, such as rational agency) should be considered a range property. There is a threshold in the scale of the relevant cognitive capacities such that all those that lie above it are to be equally considered persons for moral purposes, whereas all those that fall under it are to be equally considered as nonpersons. As I will argue in detail in Chapter 7, however, all such thresholds are ultimately arbitrary. I will defend that both the threshold view and the gradual conception of the relevance of personhood must be rejected.

Moreover, as previously discussed, the implausibility of this scenario suggests that complex cognitive capacities cannot justify attributing greater weight to the interests of those who harbor them. Possession of more complex cognitive capacities does not directly determine the extent to which individuals with a well-being of their own may be harmed or benefited by what happens to them.

Hence, if being an actual person is an irrelevant attribute that does not justify disregarding – totally or in part – the interests of those who do not qualify as such, then being a modal person is, at least, equally irrelevant. Therefore, any position that appeals to it (such as Kagan's) is equally unjustified.

2.4 Conclusion

In this chapter, I examined the concept of speciesism by committing myself to an ameliorative inquiry. Accordingly, when engaging in antispeciesist theory, "speciesism" should be reserved for the unjustified instances of disadvantageous consideration or treatment of certain individuals, either by appeal to species membership alone or to other alleged species-specific criteria.

I then examined moral anthropocentrism and distinguished it from speciesism. I claimed that they are not equivalent concepts and that the idea that anthropocentrism implies (and justifies) speciesism is unwarranted. I then provided additional reasons why anthropocentric and non-anthropocentric versions of speciesism are unjustified. Whatever the alleged species-specific attributes invoked to favor the interests of individuals of a certain species over the members of another ultimately prove morally irrelevant. Next, I argued for a categorical understanding of the concept of speciesism such that the attribution of different levels of moral considerability or degree of argumentative complexity does not alter a position's lack of justification.

Finally, I examined a position that might be construed as a further instance of speciesism – Shelly Kagan's modal personism. I conclude that even if this position were right in identifying the modal property of being a person as morally relevant, it would still not allow for a justified moral distinction between individuals based on species membership. As an account of moral considerability, personism (modal or actual) is deeply flawed and should also be rejected (a complete argument to this effect will be developed in Chapter 7).

CHAPTER 3

Wild Animal Suffering

In the previous chapter, I argued that nonhuman animals satisfy the necessary and sufficient conditions for being morally considered. I also argued that there are no sound reasons to give unequal consideration to the like interests of human and nonhuman individuals. Taking nonhuman interests into account may require different courses of action from moral agents. It may often require that we refrain from harming nonhuman animals. On other occasions, it may demand that we benefit (or help) them whenever they are in a situation of need. This includes, of course, animals living in the wild.

Many people, however, may find this conclusion hard to accept. This is because they hold an idyllic view of nature, according to which wild animals typically live good lives. Some even believe these animals have a life in "plenitude," with "plenty of time left to play."[1] Yet, as we shall see, probably what lies in store for the majority of wild animals that come into existence is a life of intense suffering and premature death. In this chapter, I examine the evidence in support of this claim. I will also argue that whatever the truth about the predominance of suffering in nature, it is still the case that many wild animals experience a tremendous amount of suffering in their lives.

3.1 Population Dynamics and Wild Animal Suffering

How much suffering is there in the wild? To examine this problem, it is not possible to directly measure the level of well-being there is in each animal's life. We do not have access to animals' mental states, and even if that were the case, it would not be possible to study *all* animals that exist in the wild. There is, however, an indirect way to assess the aggregate well-being of different animal populations. It consists in using death as a proxy

[1] jones [sic] (2014).

for suffering. There are two main reasons for accepting this proxy. First, the factors that bring about animals' death often cause them to suffer. Second, if death takes place very early in life, it is plausible that there is very little time available in an animal's life to experience something different from the process leading to their death. According to this, a crucial way of assessing the proportion of suffering in the wild is to look into wild animal population dynamics.

Population dynamics is a field of study that examines the variations of different populations of living beings through time. It can provide illuminating data for the assessment of wild animals' well-being, as it is concerned with how birth and death rates affect populations. That is, it tells us how many animals come into existence and how many of them do not survive. It also tells us when, throughout their lives, death occurs. This is a crucial point. In order to determine how well or badly animals fare in nature, it is necessary to consider both the number of deaths that take place in the wild and the length and content of a typical wild animal's life. This is relevant not only if we consider that death harms sentient individuals (see Chapter 1) but also because of the likelihood of death being preceded by suffering.

Population changes (in humans and nonhumans) have two main causes. First, migrations, which occasionally lead some individuals to leave or join a given population. Second, and most importantly, the size of populations is primarily affected by the number of births and deaths that happen over time. Populations grow when, on average, the number of animals that reach maturity and reproduce successfully outweighs the number of juvenile deaths. Populations decline when the number of born individuals that manage to become reproductive adults is lower than what is required to replace the previous generation. Populations remain stable when natality and mortality are in balance, that is, when the number of deaths roughly balances the number of births.

Thus, in an ideal situation in which a perfect substitution of individuals took place, the number of animals coming into existence in a certain population would be equal to that of the previous generation. Yet this is never the case. For each population, the number of offspring is consistently higher than the population's number of mature members. Otherwise, populations would disappear. Moreover, a typical wild animal has a much larger number of offspring than it would be required to replace them. For example, rodents can easily have more than a hundred or even several hundred offspring,[2] a bullfrog (*Rana catesbeiana*) may reach 20,000 offspring or more,[3] while a sunfish (*Mola mola*) may lay up to 300 million eggs.[4]

Certainly, if the number of individuals that come into existence and survive is higher than the number of deaths and emigration is not large enough, populations grow. This is, indeed, something that occasionally happens. For instance, since 1800, the human population has had a 7-fold increase.[5] Nevertheless, this is not what usually happens in nature, where nonhuman populations are constantly fluctuating. Their numbers may vary within certain levels, although they cannot be growing exponentially all the time. Resource availability does not allow it.[6]

We can therefore ask why wild animals commonly have such large progenies. While in the human case mortality rates have been dropping tremendously, they are extremely high in the case of most animals. For the majority of nonhuman births in nature, mortality intervenes before sexual maturity is reached.[7] This scenario is due to the reproductive strategies followed by the different species and how their growth is limited by various ecological factors.

Certain animals reproduce and transmit their genetic information to future generations by increasing the chances of each new individual to mature and reproduce. The animals that follow this strategy have few offspring and invest a great deal of parental care. Usually, they exhibit high survival rates, with many individuals reaching sexual maturity and the population stabilizing near the environment's carrying capacity (i.e., the maximum number of individuals of a certain species that the characteristics of the ecosystem allow). Typical examples include humans and the other apes, cetaceans, and other mammals such as bears and elephants, although other animals also follow that strategy, such as invertebrates like dung beetles. Most animals that live in the wild, though, follow a different reproductive strategy, which consists in producing many offspring and investing very little in parental care. As a consequence, and given the finite resources available in the environment, they have low survival rates, with most individuals dying shortly after coming into existence. Examples range

[2] Biggers et al. (1962); Wolff and Sherman (eds.) (2008).
[3] See Lu et al. (2010 [2000]). In one case a clutch of 40,000 eggs was recorded; see McAuliffe (1978).
[4] Froese and Luna (2004).   [5] Roser et al. (2013).   [6] See, for instance, Sibly and Hone (2002).
[7] Ng (1995). See also Roff. (1992); Stearns, S. C. (1992); Flatt, T. and Heyland, A. (eds.) (2011); Sæther et al. (2013).

from amphibians and fish to invertebrates and mammals, including small rodents.[8]

We can now foresee why the prevailing reproductive strategy in nature seems to increase suffering and premature death. As explained, only a minority of animals have a small number of offspring. The overwhelming majority of them have a huge number of offspring that fail to survive. Consider, for example, the case of frogs. In an average lifetime, a female frog lays many more eggs than needed to replace her and her partner. If the babies were to survive to adulthood, the population of frogs would soon be multiplied by millions. However, this is not the case. For instance, they are usually seized by predators, often freeze to death, or are killed by starvation, disease, and parasites. On average, each parent is substituted in the next generation only by one individual. As Yew-Kwang Ng remarks,

> [I]n a more or less equilibrium situation where the total population of a species is roughly stable, among the many offspring mothered by an adult female over all her life, on average not more than one female can survive to maturity to produce the next generation of offspring. Thus, from the clutch size of the species, we can have an idea as to how high is the number of those destined to starvation or to be captured.[9]

As Ng points out, animals are prevented from surviving by different causes. Some die from starvation, some are eaten by predators (often alive), and many others are killed by disease or parasites, among other causes. Thus, these animals typically die when they are very young. Due to this, their short lives appear not to contain much well-being, often ending in an excruciating death. Therefore, we have compelling reasons to believe that their lives contain much more suffering than well-being.[10] In some cases, they may even consist entirely of suffering. Since most animals that live in the wild reproduce in an aforementioned way, this implies that the majority of wild animals experience more suffering than positive well-being in their lives.[11] We have, therefore, strong reasons to conclude that on aggregate, likely predominates over well-being in the wild.

---

[8] Some species of animals combine both strategies; that is, they have a moderate number of offspring and invest some parental care.

[9] Ng (1995, pp. 270–271). By the time Ng paper was published, the idyllic view of nature had been questioned also by Mill (1969 [1874]); Gould (1994); it was also challenged at the time by Dawkins (1995).

[10] Ng (1995); Tomaisk (2015a, 2015b); Faria and Paez (2015); Horta (2017a, 2013); Fisher (2018); Alonso and Schuck-Paim (2017); Hecht (2019).

[11] To be sure, many animals that follow this reproductive strategy die when they are still not sentient, hence they do not experience any suffering at all. Nevertheless, there are many others who are indeed sentient by the time of their deaths and thus suffer throughout their short lives.

Recently, there has been some suspicion with regard to this conclusion, insofar as the model originally used by Ng seems to offer more ambiguity than it was initially presumed. According to this revision, the balance of net welfare of wild animals did not depend on a precise account of the actual evolutionary costs of suffering and well-being, of which we are vastly unsure at the moment. The alternative proposal is then to further research into refined models of animal well-being and to remain for the time being "agnostic with regard to whether total suffering will exceed enjoyment."[12]

I am sympathetic to this note of caution as well as to the call to do more research into this issue (I will elaborate on this point in Chapter 8). Yet the implications of the revision are, in my view, very limited with regard to what we ought to do. This is because opposing the harms that animals suffer in nature should not depend on whether they have lives of net suffering. Consider an analogy with the human case. When approaching so-called "human problems," we do not think that our reasons to reduce, say extreme poverty, depend on whether the set of human beings affected by extreme poverty lead net negative lives. Clearly, a state of affairs in which suffering predominates over well-being is worse than a state of affairs in which it does not. Yet, from the fact that suffering may not, or even does not, predominate it does not follow that suffering is inexistent or negligible. Suffering may not prevail in nature and still be widely spread. Suffering may not prevail in nature, and our reasons to reduce it still be very strong. We need by all means be wary of not overstating the problem but also of not understating it.

Moreover, if the crucial point of the revisionary claim is that we are unsure about the evolutionary costs of suffering and positive well-being such that we have equally strong reasons to either believe that (i) suffering exceeds well-being or that (ii) suffering does not exceed well-being, then a precautionary approach seems to require us to act as if (i) and not (ii) were the case. In the face of inconclusive evidence, the possibility of harm resultant from acting on (ii) largely exceeds the possibility of harm resultant from acting on (i). This is because acting on (i) leads to assisting individuals to the extent that we can while acting on (ii) leads to a failure of assistance. If we act on (i) and individuals have lives of net suffering, then we will level down their levels of suffering to a point in which they may be crossing the threshold to having a life worth living. If individuals do not have lives of net suffering, then we will simply level up their overall levels of well-being. Yet, if we act on (ii) and individuals have lives of net

---

[12] Groff and Ng (2019)

suffering, we will ensure they have lives not worth living by failing to reduce their suffering. If individuals do not have lives of net suffering, we will be failing to level up their overall levels of well-being. In short, acting on (i) has more expected value than acting on (ii).

Most importantly, intervention in nature would be justified even if nature turns out to contain net-positive well-being. That is, even if aggregate well-being is net positive, and even if most wild animals live net positive lives, it is still the case the most wild animals experience a tremendous amount of suffering in their lives. This remains a strong enough reason to try and find effective ways to help them.

Surely, the amount of attention put on research will be affected by how optimistic or pessimistic we are regarding the net welfare of wild animals. Yet, we would have to be implausibly optimistic in order to completely disregard wild animal suffering. Regardless of whether suffering predominates due to reproductive dynamics, wild animals (both young and adult) suffer in nature due to multiple events. In the next section, I will examine some of the most salient.

3.2 Natural Harms of Life in the Wild

It can be difficult to imagine how hard life is in nature. Wild threats to human well-being are very well established as part of human history. Although human populations, particularly those with limited assets, are still exposed to some natural hazards – mostly water scarcity and exposure to vector-borne diseases (e.g., malaria) – human societies have increasingly become less vulnerable to the impact of the natural environment. While our species has managed to reduce the impact of environmental stresses on human well-being, these are still a permanent cause of suffering and death to the majority of other animals, namely those that live in the wild.

Although human beings are seldom threatened by natural forces, on occasions, accidents occur. This is the case of unintended encounters between humans and other animals, which illustrate how terrifying life in the wild used to be and how it normally is for most animals that live there. Consider the following narration of environmentalist professor Val Plumwood, after having survived an attack from an alligator, while canoeing in Kakadu National Park, in Australia.

> Few of those who have experienced the crocodile's death roll have lived to describe it. It is, essentially, an experience beyond words of total terror (. . .) The roll was a centrifuge of boiling blackness that lasted for an eternity,

beyond endurance, but when I seemed all but finished, the rolling suddenly stopped. My feet touched bottom, my head broke the surface, and, cough-ing, I sucked at air, amazed to be alive. The crocodile still had me in its pincer grip between the legs. I had just begun to weep for the prospects of my mangled body when the crocodile pitched me suddenly into a second death roll.[13]

Humans, however, are not typically the prey of crocodiles. Being on the top of the food chain, crocodiles feed upon a wide variety of animals, ranging from crabs, prawns, fish, frogs, and insects to larger animals such as pigs, birds, reptiles, turtles, wallabies, and even other crocodiles. Death roll is a deadly attack that usually tears the prey apart so that consumption is made easier for the crocodile. Nevertheless, as in Plumwood's case, many animals manage to struggle and escape the attack, though escaping is usually not the end of their struggle to survive. They often suffer, among many other harms, serious physical injury.

a)   Physical Injury

When an animal becomes injured but not killed, they suffer at many different levels, and often the injury is so severe that it prevents her from surviving (such as when it involves mutilations). Again, Plumwood's description highlights this very common scenario:

I was alone, severely injured, and many miles from help (. . .) The left thigh hung open, with bits of fat, tendon, and muscle showing, and a sick, numb feeling suffused my entire body (. . .) Dingoes howled, and clouds of mosquitoes whined around my body. I hoped to pass out soon, but consciousness persisted. There were loud swirling noises in the water, and I knew I was easy meat for another crocodile.[14]

Without help and proper treatment, injured animals not only suffer tremendously but are also made vulnerable to considerable infections and diseases. As stated, these are excellent circumstances for making them easy targets for other predators and also conspecifics.

Most physical injuries are caused by inter- and intra-specific aggressions such as in the case of predation and territorial disputes. Very often, predators do not succeed at their attacks and the prey flees, sometimes after a long period of capture (e.g., Plumwood's case). The attack is usually performed in a sudden way, involving stressful pursuit and brutal violence

---

[13] Plumwood (1995, pp. 29–34).   [14] Ibid.

inflicted on the prey's body, causing them severe injury as a result of compression, stretching, torsion, or penetration of tissues.

In other cases, injury is caused by daily interactions with competitive conspecifics. Animals chase and fight each other for multiple purposes, such as to establish a new social or mating hierarchy or to protect the young. In addition, animals fight with other members of their own species as part of the natural strategies for survival, including competing for food, water, and space, among other resources. These aggressive behaviors usually result in injury, normally aggravated with infection and other related diseases.

Forced copulation, a particularly violent case of intraspecific aggression, can also be observed among different species of animals, namely among primates,[15] bottle-nosed dolphins,[16] and many other mammals.[17] It can also be observed in birds.[18] The rape is usually performed by immobilizing the sexually passive animal who struggles to escape and involves violent damage to bodily tissues. Among waterfowl, for example, the attack is accompanied by scalping, which results in severe injury to the head of the victim and can sometimes lead to her drowning.[19] Occasionally forced copulation is performed collectively, analogously to human "gang rape." Such is the case of "rape flights" performed by groups of ducks.[20]

Wild animals are also systematically injured by other natural events, such as flying accidents and exposure to harsh weather conditions. Impact injuries, for example, are a common cause of death among birds.[21] Chicks regularly fall down from nests and during flights birds often collide and crash in landings. As a result, animals become injured in several ways, including suffering from small bruises, hemorrhages, and fractures, especially in limbs and vertebrae.[22] Sometimes, impact injury results from hailstorms – very common, for example, among waterfowl.[23]

Crushing is also a type of injury that affects wild waterfowl[24] (as well as hedgehogs[25] and presumably many other species). As the name indicates, it takes place when an animal is pressed against the ground ("crushed"), usually by a larger animal. It is usually associated with severe hemorrhage, fracture of vertebrae, and also rupture of internal organs.

Harsh climatic conditions are also a source of injury in the wild, particularly skin burns. Skin burns are frequently due to extreme exposure

---

[15] Muller and Wrangham (2009).   [16] Connor et al. (1992).   [17] Smuts and Smuts (1993).
[18] McKinney and Evarts (1998).   [19] Ibid.   [20] Bailey et al. (1978).
[21] Beer and Ogilvie (1972).   [22] Bush (1986 [1985]).   [23] Macdonald et al. (1990).
[24] Beer and Ogilvie (1972).   [25] Bexton and Robinson (2003).

to strong sunlight[26] but are also caused by lightning strikes[27] or fires.[28] Depending on the severity of the burn, the wounds may go from minor blisters to severe tissue destruction, and in some cases may cause death. Burn wounds are definitely one of the most painful forms of injury, and they are usually aggravated by other problems such as dehydration, lethargy, and depression. In addition, wild animals sometimes get serious bruises at very low temperatures, as it is the case of frostbite, which can cause loss of limbs and damage to internal organs. (The impact of adverse climatic conditions on nonhuman well-being will be developed in a subsequent section of this chapter.)[29]

The negative impact of physical injury on wild animals' well-being is clear. It constitutes a major source of wild animal suffering. There are two ways in which this can be observed. First, directly, by considering the experience of pain associated with the wounds. And, second, indirectly, considering the disabled effects of the injury on the animal's physical performance.

Regarding the first level, injury is usually associated with intense states of pain, often accompanied by other adverse experiences of discomfort and distress. On occasions, the pain experienced by an injured animal is so excruciating that the animal struggles to get rid of the damaged area through self-mutilation.[30] The experience of pain has other negative consequences on the animal's condition, especially by leading to a decline in food and water intake. As a result, animals deal with weight loss, muscle breakdown, and impaired respiration, among other adverse effects. Most importantly, infection and disease are natural correlates of untreated injury. Without medical aid, the wounds become infected by all sorts of parasites (e.g., myiasis). This aggravates the painful situation in which the animal already is, leading to additional health complications (diarrhea, vomiting, visual disturbance, etc.).

Regarding the second level of adverse effects, a wounded debilitated animal sees them well-being jeopardized by serious injury-related disabilities. Among others, it decreases their ability to escape perilous situations and follow their conspecifics and it also prevents her from feeding and drinking properly. This debilitating condition increases the animal's susceptibility to predation, which leads to a remarkable rise in the number of deaths in the wild. As it has been thoroughly documented in the literature, predators are known to strategically prey upon substandard animals, that

[26] Schmidt (1986 [1985]).   [27] Evans (1910).   [28] Du Toit (2001).   [29] Smith (1970).
[30] Lascalles (1996).

is, those in the worst physical conditions. A well-known study carried out by a scientific team assessing the correlation between predation and substandard physical condition showed that the rate of predation of mountain lions, after an infection among the deer population, was observed to be four times higher than before the outbreak.[31]

In conclusion, physical injury is a significant threat to the well-being of animals living in the wild. It constitutes a major source of wild animal suffering. Wild animals are frequently wounded, often fatally. A significant part of this suffering could be reduced, and many deaths eventually could be prevented if only medical treatment was provided.

b) *Hunger and Thirst*

Food availability is one of the major factors limiting the growth of animal populations.[32] This is not relevant in itself to the well-being of existing wild animals. However, it does tell us something important about how the lives of these animals usually fare. Due to the reproductive strategy prevalent in nature, animals come into existence in great numbers despite the scarcity of resources. The fact that food availability is an important factor limiting the growth of animal populations implies that a vast number of wild animals typically die of starvation. Most of them die shortly after birth.[33] Others, although they survive longer, ultimately starve to death as well. It is also very common that animals that do survive suffer from malnutrition. For example, adult deer have been observed to survive even after losing as much as 25 to 30 percent of their body weight.[34]

Animals deprived of food experience a prolonged and harsh death, characterized by the progressive loss of bodily functions and by extreme distress. They suffer from severe digestive complications (such as pain in their stomach, or the excruciating states associated with constipation and diarrhea) and serious coordination problems. Other symptoms include faintness, weakness, and dizziness, accompanied by a rapid decrease in bodily temperature. In the latest stages of deprivation, animals usually fall into a coma, only to die from heart failure afterward.[35]

---

[31] Miller et al. (2008).

[32] See, for instance, Sinclair and Krebs (2002); Korpimäki et al. (2004); Prevedello et al. 2013; Anholt and Werner (1995, 1998); McNamara and Houston (1987); Sinclair and Arcese (1995); Sweitzer (1996).

[33] See, for example, Ashley et al (2020); Indiana Wildlife Disease News (2009).

[34] Michigan Department of Natural Resources (2019).   [35] Gregory (2004, p. 83).

Food availability limits the growth of animal populations in combination with other factors, as well, such as predation. In order to avoid predators, animals usually forage in areas where the probability of being preyed upon is lower. Usually, these are also places where food is scarce. When the levels of malnutrition rise to the point where there is a danger of starvation, animals risk looking for food on open plains, often crowded with predators. Thus, the number of their deaths increases.[36]

Thirst is another source of suffering and death for wild animals. As previously stated, the number of animals that exist in the wild vastly exceeds the resources available. Water is scarce, and many animals die of thirst, especially in times of drought. Thirst, by reducing blood volume, produces a feeling of permanent exhaustion, accelerates heart rate, and causes over-breathing.[37] Death is usually preceded by a period of intense dizziness and the final collapse of the animal.[38] Again, this situation is usually magnified when combined with predation. Frequently, animals under the threat of predators do not undertake the risk of seeking water. Rather they hide in secure places where they become increasingly dehydrated and eventually die of thirst. Others leave their hiding places in such a weakened condition that they become an easy prey in water-hole places. Due to their deep need of water, animals often search for fluids in food, thus managing to survive through a long period of time. Yet, as stated, food is scarce as well.[39] Thus, the norm in the wild is rather a combination of starvation and thirst, a situation that accelerates dehydration and precipitates death.

c) Extreme Weather Conditions

Weather-related events are recognizably identified as threats to human well-being. They limit food and water availability, increase exposure to disease, and isolate populations, apart from causing many other losses. In the last decade, research in global environmental change has been dealing with the question of how humans, once powerless victims of natural phenomena, may now reduce their vulnerability to them as well as prevent environmental changes from magnifying climate threats.

---

[36] Anholt and Werner (1995); McNamara and Houston (1987); Hik (1995); Horta (2010d). See also Bleicher (2017); Kohl et al. (2018).

[37] Madhavan (2004); World Preservation Foundation (2010).

[38] Kyriazakis and Tolkamp (2011); Gregory (2004).   [39] Ibid. p. 84.

Faced with the reality of wild animals living under extreme weather conditions, it does not usually come to mind that this also constitutes a serious threat to their well-being. Some people may identify extreme weather in the wild with a snowy, harmless winter to which animated films for children have accustomed us. The facts about wild animals' lives, however, contradict this belief. Extreme weather events often cause animals to massively freeze to death[40] or die of heat,[41] as well as thwarts their ability to thrive by decreasing foraging efficiency and increasing the risk of predation.[42]

Weather thus constitutes a clear source of suffering for animal populations. This is the case even when weather is compatible with feasible survival conditions. Many animals die due to extreme weather conditions, but even those that manage to survive will often suffer from cold or severe heat. This happens because the climatic conditions that make it feasible for a population to survive in the wild are not always optimal,[43] or even good, living conditions for its individual members.

To be sure, there are many cases in which this may be so, but there are also other many cases in which the reality is far from this. This happens, for instance, as animals tend to colonize the areas they can reach where, often, the environmental conditions for their survival are only barely met (including factors such as temperature or humidity levels). Since the alternative is death, animals tend to migrate to available places where life is feasible even if for most (if not all) of its members that implies living in continuous suffering. Moreover, they often migrate to places where they can live for some time and then die as a result of the extreme conditions.[44]

Ideally, animals would rather live in places where weather conditions would not only allow for survival but also ensure certain levels of well-being. That is, animals would seek places where weather-related suffering would be absent. In an ideal situation, if there were not enough resources for all, animals would simply not multiply. However, this is far from being the case in nature, where the tendency is to maximize the transmission of genes, which, as we have already seen, is not conducive to individual well-being. Finally, even in those cases in which the weather is good for the animals, climatic changes (particularly, sudden ones) can also be for them a cause of great suffering and death.[45]

---

[40] See, for example, Segelson (2010); McNulty (2010).
[41] See, for example, Garrabou et al. (2009). [42] See, for example, Conover et al. (2013).
[43] See Bowler et al. (2017) for an overview. [44] See, for example, Mott (2010).
[45] See, for example, Garrabou et al. (2009).

Some might claim that populations will finally evolve by developing adaptations to extreme weather conditions (e.g., increasing or decreasing body hair) such that suffering will be mitigated. However, this neglects the magnitude of adaptive intermediate suffering for many generations. In order for a certain trait to prevail in a given population, many individuals must fail to survive due to a lack of that trait repeatedly, generation after generation.[46] Even if the trait ultimately becomes dominant, it is only due to a massive reproductive failure of many animals in a population, which entails a vast amount of suffering and premature death.

Wild animal suffering often follows from changes in the weather. That is, the situation of wild animals may be bearable during a great part of the year but then suddenly become much worse due to a hot summer or a cold winter. In the human case, seasonal changes in the weather are usually accompanied by changes in the set of protections used to face harsh conditions (more or less clothes, heater equipment, air conditioner, etc.). On the contrary, wild animals have to face these alterations with the exact same biological equipment. As a result, many animals that might thrive during a great part of the year may not be able to survive due to extreme temperatures and usually end up dying in agonizing ways.[47] Seasonal suffering hence leads to a high death rate in the wild and, sometimes, may even result in the extinction of a given population.[48] However, for the reasons already stated, this is not very different from when populations thrive, which imply that most of their members die shortly after birth. In addition, the scale of suffering is intensified once we realize that even if an extinction takes place, animals will tend to colonize that area again, leading to a continuous cycle of suffering, death, and recolonization.[49]

Finally, extreme climate phenomena such as floods, droughts, heavy snows, or heat waves have a tremendous impact on wild animals' lives. Exposure to cold can cause death and injury to animals. In addition, it requires a great caloric intake of food, usually scarce when these natural events take place. For example, in a heavy snow, grazing animals may be deprived of reaching food and water and may die from hypothermia or starvation.[50] Weather-related events are also a cause of disease in wild animals, sometimes being responsible for huge epidemics.[51] This has been particularly linked to the transmission of vector-borne diseases, observed as

---

[46] Brown and Brown (1998).
[47] White (2008). See also, for example, Salzman (1982); DelGiudice et al. (2002); Berger et al. (2004).
[48] Thomas et al. (1996); Parmesan et al. (2000).   [49] Dias (1996); Battin (2004).
[50] Conover et al. (2013).   [51] Ytrehus et al. (2008).

a major cause of mortality in different species of afflicted wild animals, including rabbits[52] and amphibians.[53]

The situation of wild animals is sometimes aggravated by other weather-dependent factors, which play a significant role in wild animals' well-being. For example, some animals depend on certain levels of humidity to survive. Again, it may be feasible for some animals to survive in places where humidity is barely above the survival threshold.[54] However, these animals will suffer extremely in these conditions. In addition, some levels of precipitation, even if not relevant for survival concerns, may have a very negative impact on the psychology of some animals.

In sum, wild animals are exposed to extreme climate and weather conditions, which directly and indirectly constitute a huge threat to their well-being.

d) Psychological Stress

In 1936, during an experiment carried out on rats, Hans Selye observed that individuals from the control group, in spite of having been exposed only to placebo agents, were showing the exact same physiological changes as the rats from the experimental group (ulcers, atrophy of the immune system, and enlargement of adrenaline glands). He then hypothesized that what animals were responding to was the common unpleasant experience both groups were going through. Selye chose a term previously used in engineering to describe the way the rats' bodies were responding to the negative impact they were suffering. He called it stress and thus initiated the field of stress physiology.[55]

The effects of psychological stress on nonhuman animals have been the object of what now amounts to a considerable body of scientific research. This is the case due precisely to the physiological similarities between human and nonhuman animals,[56] the latter constituting an enlightening (and allegedly ethical) source of data that helps us explain relevant phenomena about the former[57] – the impact of psychological stress on human health being one of them.[58]

Stress is the physiological response to a stimulus (called "stressor") that is perceived by animals as a harmful event or a threat to their survival. The response may be triggered by an actual environmental pressure, such as

---

[52] Henning et al. (2005).   [53] See Berger et al. (2004); Pounds et al. (2006).
[54] Ludwig (1945).   [55] Sapolszky (1990).   [56] Ferdowsian and Merskin (2012).
[57] Ottenweller (2000).   [58] See, for instance, Biondi and Zannino (1997); Verbitski et al. (2020).

extreme weather conditions (physical stressor), or by the mere expectation that a threat is about to take place (psychological stressor). It increases the discharge of adrenaline and cortisol (the so-called "stress hormones"), leading to a rise in heart rate and blood pressure. It also temporarily suppresses various biological processes, such as the immune system. The alteration of immune functions can in turn impair the individual's health in various ways, thereby increasing morbidity to disease and infection. As in humans, stress can often cause arrhythmias and heart attacks, which may sometimes be lethal.[59]

Nonhuman animals are afflicted by an enormous variety of stressors. However, the effects of the adverse circumstances animals face daily in the wild are still an undeveloped topic of scientific inquiry. Most research that has been carried out to date either deals with the effects of psychological stress on domestic animals[60] or with the effects of housing on wild animals in captivity.[61]

Wild animals, however, go through very stressful situations in their natural environments. For example, they experience physical trauma, live in places with a high density of predators or parasites, face conflicts with conspecifics, and have to endure constant variations of food, water, and temperature. In addition to how harmful in themselves these situations can be for animals, they also cause them to suffer from psychological stress.

Predator-induced stress is the most salient form of stress in the wild, with research showing that it can have long-lasting effects on wild animals' psychology and behavior.[62] It is usually triggered by three main events: (i) predatory activity, (ii) predator-avoidance decision-making, and (iii) the expectation of predation.

Regarding (i), stress responses are caused by the scenario in which a prey engages in direct confrontation with a predator. The capture, which often results in the prey's death, is usually preceded by the experience of intense terror that comes with fleeing for one's life. The path that leads to death often involves brutal fighting for survival, and it is not uncommon for the horror of the event to be intensified by the prey being consumed while still alive. The encounter between an animal and her predator may be so intense that sometimes stress alone can kill the prey.[63] As an example, in

---

[59] See Fink (2016), for an overview.
[60] See, for example, Dantzer and Mormède (1983); Wiepkema and van Adrichem (eds.) (1987); Moberg and Mench (2000); Broom and Johnson (1993); Ahmed-Farid (2021).
[61] See, for example, Price (1999); Dickens et al. (2009); Carlstead et al. (1993); Clubb and Mason (2003).
[62] Zanette (2020). [63] McCauley et al. (2011).

a study carried out on wild rats, after being forced to listen to a tape recording of a fight between a cat and a rat, some animals died of a heart attack.[64]

Regarding (ii), stress is significantly correlated with predator-avoidance decision-making. That is, with the forced balance animals have to make between food availability and predator density. Given both environmental stressors, animals must choose either to decrease food intake or to increase the risk of being caught by predators.[65] Both options imply great levels of stress for animals, though they typically favor foraging less over being exposed to predators. Animals decrease the risk of predation by hiding in places where food is scarce, but the likelihood of predators is low. In such circumstances, additional stressors arise, mostly due to starvation and dehydration.

Regarding (iii), the expectation of predation is a powerful psychological stressor for wild animals. It is sometimes aggravated by certain human interventions in the wild, such as ecosystem restoration programs involving the reintroduction of predators. The process usually goes as follows: A certain species is transforming the ecosystem in a certain way, and its ancient predator, currently extinct in that ecosystem, is reintroduced in order to restore the ecosystem to the way it previously was. By doing so it is expected that the predators will stop their prey from changing the ecosystem both by killing them and by changing their behavior. This happens, for example, in the case of the reintroduction of wolves in areas in which deer graze a plant over certain limits considered to be acceptable. The wolves are reintroduced to stop the deer from grazing in certain areas. They will prey upon the deer, thereby reducing their numbers, and, in particular, because the deer will stop grazing openly out of their fear of being killed by the wolves. As already stated, when confronted with the risk of predation, animals choose to decrease foraging by hiding in more scarce places where predators cannot easily locate them. The biological dynamics that follow from this is usually referred to as the "ecology of fear."[66] A very representative case of this type of harmful human intervention is the reintroduction of wolves that took place at Yellowstone Park in the United States, which halved the population of deer.[67] Apart from living in a "landscape of fear," these animals are also prone to suffer from other related complications caused by food and water scarcity and usually die in very painful ways, stricken by disease and other afflictions.

[64] Gregory (2004, p. 18).   [65] Clinchy et al. (2004).   [66] Bleicher (2017); Kohl et al.(2018).
[67] Laundré (2001). See Horta (2010d) for criticisms.

Apart from predation-induced stress, other stressors in the wild have been recognized in the literature such as stress responses to weather,[68] food shortages,[69] and drought.[70] All species in the wild are likely to suffer from these environmental pressures. Other pressures, however, only affect a small range of wild animals, namely species that exhibit social behavior. Life in social groups, in which competition and conflict govern daily interactions, involves great costs for animals. The social status that each animal occupies in a given dominant hierarchy may have a tremendous impact on their well-being. For example, different social species like primates,[71] monkeys,[72] rodents,[73] and fish[74] have exhibited stress responses to social subordination. This situation has been shown to have an impact on reproductive competence as well as to be related to depression in different low-ranking members of social species.[75] It also increases the susceptibility of these animals to stress-related diseases.[76] In social species, serious episodes of stress are also triggered by adverse events such as maternal separation, for both mother and child. This separation may have profound consequences on the physiology and behavior of these animals, often throughout their entire lives. After the separation, infants exhibit increased reactivity to stress across their lifespans, and the risk of disease becomes higher. Rodents and primates[77] are common victims of this form of suffering, though there are no good reasons to believe it is not widespread among other social species. Mothers, once separated, show diverse sickness behaviors.[78]

As these facts show, psychological stress constitutes a form of suffering to which animals living in the wild are constantly exposed. Fear, anxiety, and distress can be a part of their lives as much as they can be a part of human experience.

e) Predation

As illustrated by Plumwood's *experience of being a prey*, human beings are not immune to attacks from predators. Although human vulnerability to predation is exceptionally low when compared to other animals, in some parts of the planet deaths still occur. In Namibia, for instance, crocodiles killed 23 people between 2000 and 2004[79] and statistics for the year

---

[68] Romero et al. (2000).   [69] Kitaysky et al. (1999).   [70] Sapolsky (1986).
[71] Abbott et al. (2003).   [72] Shiverly et al. (1997).
[73] Koolhas et al. (1997); Koolhas et al. (1997).   [74] Fox et al. (1997).   [75] Sapolsky (2005).
[76] Sapolsky (2004).   [77] Pryce et al. (2002).   [78] Hennessy et al. (2001).
[79] See Table 4 of Republic of Namibia (2004).

2015 alone report 58 fatal attacks in the African continent.[80] From 1990 to 2004 in Tanzania, there have been 815 lion attacks on humans, from which 563 terminated in death.[81] Also, in the Indian state of Kashmir, leopards were responsible for the killing of 16 people from 2005 to 2007.[82] The terror of dying at the claws of a predator may be hardly conceivable for most of us humans. Yet, for almost the totality of wild animals, it constitutes a daily threat.

Predation is a biological interaction between two organisms that results in the killing and consumption of one of them (the prey) by the other (the predator). The predatory activity may assume distinct forms. For example, the prey may be consumed after or prior to being killed. The killing may be abrupt or rather slow and agonizing. Nevertheless, it consistently involves great violence being inflicted on the prey. Since all nonhuman animals at some point in their lives are exposed to predators, predation proves to be one of the most significant sources of wild animal suffering.

The presence of predators in a given environment limits the size of prey populations in two main ways. First, it directly impacts the prey population mortality rates through successful predatory interactions. Many people believe that there is a perfect balance between predator and prey populations such that no significant variations in their size take place throughout time. However, the biological dynamics that result from predator–prey interactions typically constitute a cycle of growth and decline for both predator and prey populations, even in relatively stable environments. A prey population will tend to reproduce and grow exponentially until it is limited by predation. This means that the population will decrease while the number of predators grows. Then predators will ultimately surpass their food supply and end up starving.[83] Thus, predator population will also decrease. As the number of predators declines, the prey population will increase again. The cycle shall then indefinitely repeat itself.[84]

Second, the presence of predators indirectly restrains population numbers by being associated with other harmful events such as starvation and psychological stress. This happens mostly due to the creation of the so-called "landscape of fear" (as already discussed in previous sections by

---

[80] Sideleau (2016).   [81] Packer et al. (2005).   [82] Nabi et al. (2009).

[83] Other factors may also affect this dynamic of suffering and death both in prey and predator populations, such as competition among predators, other prey available, lack of food or water, and weather conditions, among others.

[84] See, for instance, the paradigmatic case of prey–predator interactions between lemmings and stoats; Gilg et al. (2003).

which animals reduce the risk of meeting predators by staying away from open places where food is normally available). This situation commonly leads to permanent malnourishment of prey populations and often leads to death by starvation. The permanent situation of alarm in which animals encounter themselves is also responsible for triggering intense stress responses (in line with what has been described in the previous section).

Predation is a powerful selecting force in nature, both for prey and predator species. Species usually hunted as prey have developed different types of defenses such as coloration, camouflage, and mimicry,[85] by which they avoid or resist attacks. Predator species, in turn, have also evolved in a variety of ways so as to increase predatory success. Some adaptations include speed,[86] camouflage,[87] and an advanced sensorial system.[88] As regards specific killing adaptations, they include sharp teeth and claws, venom release, and strong jaws.[89] Mimicry, long identified with the chemical defense technique by which the prey tries to look like another species in order to survive, has recently been observed in some feline species as a hunting technique. Researchers in the Brazilian Amazon discovered that margays, a species of wild cats, imitate the vocal sounds of tamarin monkeys in order to attract them to what they are lead to believe is a conspecific and ultimately kill them.[90] The process by which all these traits become prevalent is built upon the suffering and death of those countless individuals (both predator and prey) who failed to adapt to their environment.

It is difficult to estimate the suffering that results from being preyed upon. Nevertheless, a brief overview of the different killing methods that animals use in the wild may help us imagine how the experience of being a prey must feel. There is a widespread belief that attacks by predators happen in a rather fast and elegant way. Nature documentaries usually reinforce this mistaken view of death in the wild. Contrary to this, though, being preyed upon is usually a terribly bloody experience that involves struggling desperately for survival, often for many hours. Consider the following case of a baby elephant being eaten alive by hyenas, documented by the photographer Michael Poliza:

> This scene is probably the most shocking and emotionally difficult scene I have ever witnessed in nature. This young elephant got stuck in mud and was abandoned by his parents. Hyenas found it and started to eat it alive.

[85] Stevens (2007).   [86] Bro-Jørgensen (2013).   [87] Pembury Smith and Ruxton (2020).
[88] Galloway et al. (2020).   [89] Biknevicius and Van Valkenburgh (2019).
[90] Dell'Amore (2010).

The calf could obviously not move and the hyenas started at the trunk and ate it and most of the head skin and meat (. . .) We only found the elephant at a time when the trunk was already eaten and I could only "handle" to take a few photographs. At this stage it was already too late for the calf. But it did not let go (. . .) About 2 hours later the elephant was still alive and at that time the hyenas had already eaten the eyes and skinned his skull completely. The calf kept fighting and continuously called for help.[91]

It is characteristic of hyenas to eat their prey while they are still alive. This may not be as surprising as it may be regarding other mammals that enjoy a better reputation in the wild (at least as we see it). Chimpanzees, for example, not typically represented as predators, can also exhibit predatory behavior. The way in which chimpanzees hunt small monkeys by chasing, capturing, and ripping them apart is particularly appalling.[92] On occasions, they may hunt other animals as well:

At 1125 on 16 December 1981 (Case 34), four adult male chimpanzees surrounded and captured a large juvenile bushpig and began to eat its hindlimbs, while the piglet was still alive and struggling to free itself. They looked puzzled with the piglet's struggle for life, and it seemed to be difficult for them to kill the piglet. At 1139, NT (alpha male) struck the piglet with his elbow several times, eventually killing it; it took at least 15 min for the piglet to die. At 1306, NT intermittently struck the dead piglet's head with his elbow and back of his hand for 9 min.[93]

Some male orcas are known to chase humpback whales and their calves to exhaustion so that they can prey upon the unprotected calf,[94] mostly for their soft tongues.[95] The same "endurance–exhaustion" technique has been observed in whale predation on bluefin tuna.[96] Other particularly gruesome forms of predation carried out by large mammals include wolves disemboweling their prey, coyotes chasing and biting the legs of the prey until they collapse, felines or cougars killing their prey by suffocation, and bears mauling and biting the spine of the prey for long periods of time before killing.

Some of the most terrifying predators can be found among reptiles. Snakes, for example, usually swallow the prey whole and alive. The prey then becomes immobilized by venom injected through the fangs until the digestive process takes place. Another deadly carnivorous reptile is the Komodo dragon, which follows a "venom-plus-wounding" approach to their prey. Due to their very sharped teeth, these animals combine venom

---

[91] Poliza (2002).   [92] See, for instance, Takahata et al. (1984).   [93] Ibid., p. 123.
[94] Pitman et al. (2015).   [95] Jefferson et al. (1991).   [96] Guinet et al. (2007).

discharges with multiple lacerations on the victim.[97] This always results in a certain death, even if the prey manages to escape the attack. Small mammals such as shrews also carry out a similar predatory technique, by paralyzing and slowly devouring their prey, sometimes for days, until the animal finally dies due to their injuries.[98]

Invertebrates also sometimes hunt and kill other animals in ways that cause them great amounts of pain. Birds, snakes, frogs, lizards, mice, and bats are common prey of spiders, for example. Usually, the process is long since it consists in a smaller animal eating a much bigger one. Spiders may discharge venom into the prey or inject them with other substances that cause the liquidification of internal organs and then consume them.[99] On other occasions, the prey becomes trapped on the webs and ultimately dies of exhaustion, lack of food or liquids, or excessive temperatures. Insects can also hunt and kill their prey in very painful ways. Some beetles are a paradigmatic example of an extremely long predatory attack. They paralyze the prey and feed off the animal for many hours until they die.[100]

Finally, predation is more prevalent than we usually think of; it only needs an opportunity to arise. Animals such as turtles, fishes,[101] and frogs have been recorded eating mice. In addition, animals can also be trapped and eaten by carnivorous plants. These plants (e.g., *Nepenthes*) normally have a deep cavity with chemicals used to trap their victims (mostly insects but also small vertebrates), from where it is almost impossible to escape. Usually, the prey drowns and gets consumed by the plant.[102]

From what has been said, it follows that predation is, perhaps more vividly than any other natural event, a major source of wild animal suffering and death.

f) Parasitism and Disease

Other naturally destructive events sometimes associated with predation, though often overlooked as a cause of wild animal suffering, are parasitism and parasitoidism. They consist in an interaction between two organisms that usually takes place during long periods of time (unlike predation) by which one organism lives and feeds upon the other (the host), thereby reducing their fitness (i.e., individual capacity to successfully reproduce and survive) and ultimately leading to their death. Parasites and parasitoids

---

[97] Boyd et al. (2021).   [98] Kowalski and Rychlik (2018).
[99] See, for example, Malli et al. (1999); Wigger et al. (2002).   [100] Wizen and Gasith (2011).
[101] Kelly et al. (2016).   [102] Chin et al. (2010); Clarke et al. (2009).

have a similar life history insofar as they spend most of their existence obtaining nourishment from a host. Parasites, unlike parasitoids, do not kill their host although the association has a negative impact on the host's fitness.

Parasites and parasitoids (henceforth only "parasites") may live inside the body of their host, feeding on internal organs and reproducing profusely, such as is the case of helminths (flatworms) and protozoa (unicellular organisms). The life cycle of these parasites varies significantly, insofar as they use different strategies for survival, which consist in moving from one host to another. Helminths, for example, which usually infect the host by being ingested, normally reside in the host's gastrointestinal tract, where they release their offspring. These, by being then excreted, will eventually find another host in the environment who will later harbor them. Protozoa, on the other hand, can be found in the host's blood system. In order to reach another host, they usually require the assistance of vector insects, who, through biting and sucking the host's blood, carry the parasite from one animal to another.[103] Alternatively, parasites may be located on the surface of the host's body, usually on their skin or fur, as it is typical of ticks and mites. These external parasites usually travel between hosts when they make direct contact.

Throughout the lifetime of wild animals, they may become the host of multiple parasites.[104] Being the host of a parasite affects animals in various harmful ways. Parasites have been known to cause behavioral alterations on their hosts so as to significantly enhance transmission, primarily by increasing their vulnerability to predators[105] (the final hosts in their life-cycle). *Toxoplasma Gondii*, for example, a protozoan parasite, is widespread among wild mammals and birds, though mostly harbored by felids. This parasite has been reported to manipulate a rat's (intermediate host) perception to the risk of being preyed upon by cats (final host).[106] Another example consists in a flatworm that infects fish and induces cataract formation so that the fish's ability to escape bird predators is impaired.[107] The green-banded broodsac, arguably one of the most morbid forms of helminths, enters into the digestive system of snails and grows large cysts

---

[103] For the specific differences between helminths and protozoa, see, for instance, Soulsby (1982); Jameson et al. (2018).

[104] It has been estimated, although not completely settled yet, that the number of parasites that exists in the wild is overwhelming, outstripping four times the number of host species. See Zimmer (2003).

[105] Hudson et al. (1992); Thomas et al. (2010); Hatcher et al. (2014); Sures et al. (2017).

[106] Berdoy et al. (2000).   [107] Seppälä et al. (2004).

that travel to the host's tentacles, giving them the appearance of a cater-
pillar and thus increasing their exposure to bird predators.[108]

Parasites also harm their hosts in more direct forms. Population declines
in threatened mammals have been associated with the presence of up to
30 species of parasites. This threat is estimated to affect 54 percent of the
carnivorous population and 67 percent of primates.[109] Among other mammals, several parasites are also associated with high death rates, usually
aggravated by a combination of food deprivation and other diseases. The
canine sarcoptic mite, for example, widespread in cats, pigs, horses, and
many other species, has been identified as the cause of up to 90 percent
mortality of the fox population in Norway and Sweden and since then
reported in other places across Europe.[110]

Even when parasitism does not result in death, the damage to the host's
body is significant. Leishmania, for example, transmitted to wild canids by
the bite of sandflies, leads to leprosy-like lesions to the nose and mouth.[111]
Giardia lamblia, a protozoan parasite common among beavers,[112] various
mammals,[113] and waterfowl[114] and acquired by the accidental ingestion of
cysts from feces of infected animals, has nasty effects on its host, such as
chronic diarrhea, abdominal cramps, nausea, dehydration, and weight loss.
Wild birds, highly susceptible to harbor parasites, are usually damaged
by different types of destructive worms. They often exhibit large
visible tunnels on the stomach or intestine, with bacterial peritonitis and
secondary infections as well as thick-walled granuloma.[115] In addition, birds
are also prone to host tracheal worms, which results in major respiratory
distress, against which they struggle by coughing, sneezing, and shaking their
heads in an attempt to expel the parasites. As a consequence, they may lose
body mass, suffer from anemia, and often die of starvation.[116] Moreover, all
infected animals see their reproductive success impaired by the general
debilitating condition caused by harboring parasites.[117]

Some particularly rare and gruesome forms of parasitism may also be
found in the wild. Consider the infection by cordyceps (*Ophiocordyceps
unilateralis*), a particularly horrifying parasite fungus that affects wild ant
populations. After infecting the host, the fungus takes control over her
nervous system, a process also known as zombification. The ant is directed

[108] Robinson (1947).   [109] Pedersen et al. (2007).   [110] Simpson (2002).
[111] Font et al. (1996); Kaszak et al. (2015).   [112] Dixon et al. (1997).   [113] Adam (2001).
[114] Graczyk et al. (1998).   [115] Cole and Friend (1999).   [116] Ibid.
[117] Hillegass et al. (2010); Hu et al. (2008).

to a location where the fungus can continue its life cycle, such as the underside of a leaf. Once there, the fungus forces the host to grip the leaf with their mandibles, thereby fixing their in place. The fungus eats the ant tissue and replaces it with fungal sprouts, out of which spores shall be finally released.[118]

As any other limiting factor for populations, parasitism has been observed to interact with other environmental stressors, such as inclement conditions[119] and food availability, thereby worsening its effects on wild animals.[120] For instance, birds parasitized with blowfly larvae had a higher mortality rate than unparasitized individuals during a period of wet, cold weather.[121] Likewise, snowshoe hares have exhibited the presence of intestinal parasites only during periods of food scarcity.[122]

Wild animals may also suffer from parasitic diseases caused by bacteria. Among the most prevalent are Tuberculosis – a disease predominantly affecting the lungs and reported in various wild species (including badgers, foxes, and rats[123]) – and Lyme disease, considered one of the most important tick-borne diseases, which affects vital organs such as the heart and nervous system. It has been observed in a wide range of species such as birds, squirrels, various rodents, and deer.[124]

One of the most startling instances of parasitic diseases is the Devil Facial Tumor Disease, responsible for a 60 percent decline of the Tasmania Devil population. It consists of a highly transmissible parasitic cancer, caused by a nonviral clone of malignant cells.[125] The transmission occurs through biting, a very common activity among the devils, by which the hosts infect other devils. As a result, a multiplicity of complications arise, such as a failure in properly feeding due to tumors and metastases in the oral cavity, as well as various infections. Death usually follows long periods of acute pain and starvation.[126] Currently, wombats are being

---

[118] See, for instance, Hywel-Jones (1996); Evans (2011). There are many other zombifying parasites that alter the behavior of their hosts by controlling their minds. Extreme manipulations of behavior include causing hosts to chase their natural predators (e.g., one parasite causes mice to feel attracted to cats that eat them acquiring the parasite; another causes fish to swim toward the surface where they are eaten by birds; others cause animals that normally live in dark unexposed places to lose eyesight and so to seek the light where there are seen by predators), or causing aggressive behavior leading to attacks that help the parasite spread. For a detailed description, see Zimmer (2003, Chapter 3). Some even cause hosts to commit suicide with the body destruction aiding the spread of the parasite. See, for instance, Libersat et al. (2009).

[119] Howe (1992). [120] Chapman et al. (2006). [121] Wobeser (2013). [122] Murray (1998). [123] Corner (2006). [124] Simpson (2002). [125] Australian Geographic (2012). [126] See R. Loh et al. (2006). Pyecroft et al. (2007); McCallum et al. (2007).

decimated by a parasitic mite – sarcoptic mange – which literally eats the animals alive.[127]

Diseases in the wild are very harmful to wild animals' well-being, leading them to an early and painful death. Nevertheless, they are usually very hard to detect. Their prevalence among wild animals can be compared to an iceberg. It is only its top that appears visible to us, an insignificant fraction of its total volume. There are two main causes that converge to bring about this scenario. First, until very recently, research on wild animal disease has been an underestimated field of inquiry. Wild animal disease is thought to be relevant only inasmuch as it proves instrumental in bettering our knowledge about and treatment of diseases affecting human and domestic animal populations.[128] Second, disease is a fundamentally surreptitious phenomenon, often resulting from many factors interacting simultaneously. Unlike humans and other animals under human control, wild animals are anonymous. We can make estimations about their numbers and whereabouts, but we do not have accurate records of them. In addition, sick and dead animals are very quickly assimilated into the environment by predators and scavengers. As a consequence, the results of wild animal death caused by disease remain, for the most part, hidden from us.[129] This strongly suggests that the number of animals affected by disease and the magnitude of the suffering and death that follows from it are much greater than we normally think of.

Disease in wild animals is generated by a causal network consisting in several factors that interact to produce it. Along with the infectious agents, many environmental factors may contribute to reducing immune responses, such as overcrowding, exposure to predators, food availability, and inclement weather. Conversely, disease may indirectly affect the survival of wild animals through increased vulnerability to other factors such as predation, nutrition, and harsh weather conditions.[130] Since animals need to allocate

[127] Old, J. M., Sengupta, C., Narayan, E., & Wolfenden, J. (2018). Sarcoptic mange in wombats – A review and future research directions. *Transboundary and Emerging Diseases*, 65(2), 399–407. Martin, A. M., Burridge, C. P., Ingram, J., Fraser, T. A., & Carver, S. (2018). Invasive pathogen drives host population collapse: Effects of a travelling wave of sarcoptic mange on bare-nosed wombats. *Journal of Applied Ecology*, 55(1), 331–341. Stannard, H. J., Wolfenden, J., Hermsen, E. M., Vallin, B. T., Hunter, N. E., & Old, J. M. (2020). Incidence of sarcoptic mange in bare-nosed wombats (Vombatus ursinus). *Australian Mammalogy*, 43(1), 85–95.

[128] Nevertheless, information on the existence of certain diseases in wild animals is now increasingly being collected by different organizations such as the National Wildlife Health Center in the United States or the Canadian Cooperative Wildlife Health Centre in Canada, among others.

[129] In a study carried out on ducks killed by botulism, only 7 percent of the carcasses were recovered. See Stzutenbaker et al. (1986).

[130] Kavaliers and Colwell (1995); Ives and Murray (1997).

finite physiological resources among these competing needs, those resources used to prevent or fight disease will be displaced from reproduction, predator avoidance, or endurance of inclement conditions, creating a disadvantage for sick animals within their populations.

Wild animals also suffer and die due to diseases typically associated with human beings. Malaria, for instance, a vector-borne disease still widespread across human populations around the world, affects a broad spectrum of wild animals, ranging from primates[131] to birds, including penguins.[132] It has been claimed that Ebola, one of the most contagious viral diseases, has been responsible in the last decades for the death of approximately one-third of the gorilla and chimpanzee populations around the world.[133] Other examples include hepatitis B, which can be found in a variety of mammals and birds, such as chimpanzees[134] or ducks.[135] A particularly shocking case of disease that affects wild animals while having been long eradicated in human populations is the Black Death, found in prairie dogs and ferrets. The disease has decimated the population of prairie dogs in North America, and, as a result, black-foot ferrets, their natural predators, have also been affected.[136] Other well-known diseases among domesticated animals, such as swine fever and brucellosis, also affect wild populations. In Europe, the swine fever was responsible for the death of over 10,000 pigs back in 1997 and can still be found in wild boars.[137] In Yellowstone, for example, buffalos have manifested a high vulnerability to brucellosis.[138]

As it has been shown, animals in the wild are prone to be infected by a large number of parasites. They are also highly susceptible to other different forms of disease. In the overwhelming majority of cases, these conditions either cause huge suffering to the animals or are responsible for bringing about their deaths by direct or indirect means, that is, by increasing their susceptibility to predation and other harmful events.

3.3 A Minimal Case for Intervention

In the previous chapter, I argued that the interests of animals that live in the wild should be given a consideration equal to the interests of other sentient individuals. Sometimes, considering their interests requires that we refrain from harming them. Some other times, those interests call for

---

[131] Prugnolle et al. (2010, 2013).   [132] Fix et al. (1988).   [133] Torres (2012).
[134] Hu et al. (2000).   [135] Marion et al. (1984).   [136] Leggett (2009).
[137] Godfroid and Käsbohrer (2002).   [138] Buffalo Field Campaign (2016).

our intervention in order to alleviate animal suffering or, alternatively, to provide animals with some good.

Intervening in nature would not be of foremost concern if the idyllic view of nature were true. Nonetheless, as I have explained throughout this chapter, nature is not a source of well-being for animals. Instead, it is a source of permanent suffering and death.

First, data from population dynamics show that due to the prevalent reproductive strategy in nature, animal suffering likely outweighs positive well-being. For the majority of these animals, their average situation is actually analogous to a case of massive extinction. A population becomes extinct when all its members die. Often, all of its members die in misery; that is, they experience tremendously painful deaths. Yet this scenario is quite similar to the one that takes place when populations thrive, which, as stated, does not imply that its members do flourish but rather implies that most of its members have short lives, full of suffering, ending in an agonizing death. Only a small minority of wild animals (those who survive) experience something different from what happens in a scenario of extinction.

Second, during their lives, wild animals face many threats to their health and physical integrity, which entail a great amount of suffering: physical injury, severe hunger and thirst, extreme weather conditions, and psychological stress. In addition, they experience excruciating deaths due to predation or parasitism, often debilitated and killed by disease.

The evidence thus suggests that we have strong reasons to intervene in nature in order to reduce wild animal suffering. On the face of it, this conclusion may seem counterintuitive. Nonetheless, when considering similar cases involving human beings, our intuitions become adjusted. Consider, again, Val Plumwood's crocodile attack, to which I have been referring throughout the chapter. The fact that she was able to tell her story indicates something of crucial importance – that she obtained help and survived:

> In the end, I was found in time and survived against many odds. A similar combination of good fortune and human care enabled me to overcome a leg infection that threatened amputation or worse.[139]

Most of us think that Plumwood was fortunate to survive. We also think that those who helped her did the right thing. As we are aware, wild animals' encounters with predators and other natural causes of injury often have a very different end. However, if human and nonhuman suffering is to be equally considered, there are no non-arbitrary considerations that

---

[139] Plumwood (1995, pp. 29–34).

favor assisting Plumwood and not assisting other animals in similar circumstances. We ought to act so as to alleviate the suffering of other individuals, and we must do so while rejecting all kinds of unjustified differential considerations of those in need.

That is indeed how in the previous chapters I argued that we should proceed. I presented several arguments that show that is unjustified and that we must take the interests of all sentient animals (including animals that live in the wild) into full moral consideration. If those arguments are correct, then we have reasons to alleviate the suffering experienced by all sentient animals. Notice that even if speciesism is correct, as long as the interests of animals matter to some extent, we would still have reasons to aid those who are in need of help in nature. The fact that animals that live in the wild endure numerous and permanent harms is then relevant in order to determine the kind of environmental interventions that are morally due.

The minimal case for intervention in nature can thus be synthesized as follows. On the assumption that

(1)   We ought to aim at preventing or reducing the harms suffered by other individuals, whenever it is in our power to do so.

If

(2)   All sentient individuals, including nonhuman animals, are fully morally considerable

and

(3)   The interests of wild animals are systematically frustrated by different natural events,

then

(4)   We have reasons to intervene in nature so as to prevent that wild animals have lives of net suffering or, at least, to reduce their suffering, whenever it is in our power to do so.

The minimal case for intervention in nature is based primarily on plausible moral claims (1) and (2) and on facts about wild animal suffering (3). It is compatible with most plausible normative positions (at least, with those that accept the existence of positive obligations) and can therefore attract wide support. I will deal with this in the conclusion of the book. For now, the next chapters will be dedicated to assessing the different objections that can be pressed against intervening in nature for the benefit of wild animals.

CHAPTER 4

Perversity and Futility

In the previous chapter, I provided an account of the different harmful events that wild animals have to endure and of the causes of the likely prevalence of suffering over well-being in nature. I claimed that, in light of the evidence presented and the arguments advanced in the previous chapters, we have decisive reasons to intervene in nature in order to reduce these harms. Yet several objections may be put forward against the conclusion that intervening is what we should do.

Certain positions would claim that

(I) *we have decisive reasons not to intervene.* That is, the reasons we have not to intervene in nature are stronger than the reasons we may have to intervene. Thus, not intervening is what we have most reason to do. The facts that give us decisive reasons not to intervene may vary, depending on the position one endorses. For example, it may be that intervention would *jeopardize* other more important values, it would have *perverse* effects, or it would simply be *futile*. If this were the case, then not intervening would be what we ought to do.

Other positions would endorse a different claim, according to which

(II) *we have merely sufficient reasons not to intervene.* That is, the reasons we have not to intervene in nature are not outweighed by the reasons we may have to intervene. There may be several explanations of why our reasons not to intervene are merely sufficient. For example, it may be that we normally lack the kind of relationship with wild animals that generates decisive reasons to help them. Thus, our reasons for and against intervention are equally strong. This does not imply that we should not intervene, but rather that intervening is not what we ought to do.

In this and the following chapters, I assess the different objections that can be pressed against intervening in nature for the benefit of wild animals.

First, I develop a taxonomy that classifies these objections not by their axiological assumptions but by the strength of the reasons there are not to intervene; and, in a more specific way, by the particular type of criticism aimed at intervention. Second, after assessing each of the alleged categories of reasons on which to base the case against intervention, I claim that (i) it is false that we have decisive reasons not to intervene and (ii) it is also false that our reasons to intervene are merely sufficient. This is because the reasons we have to intervene prove to be stronger than the reasons we may have not to do so.

4.1 Objections to Intervention: A Taxonomy

In his 1991 book *The Rhetoric of Reaction*, Albert O. Hirschman[1] describes the conservative opposition to progressive social change as consisting of three principal reactive-reactionary theses: (1) the *perversity* thesis, (2) the *futility* thesis, and (3) the *jeopardy* thesis. He writes,

> According to the *perversity* thesis, any purposive action to improve some feature of the political, social or economic order only serves to exacerbate the condition one wishes to remedy. The *futility* thesis holds that attempts at social transformation will be unavailing, that they will simply fail "to make a dent." Finally, the *jeopardy* thesis argues that the cost of the proposed change is too high as it endangers some previous, precious accomplishment.[2]

We can reformulate the previous theses as follows:

(1) *Perversity*: Action x will have consequences opposite to those intended.
(2) *Futility*: Action x will have none of the intended consequences whatsoever.
(3) *Jeopardy*: Action x will threaten other important values.

A review of the common arguments against intervening in nature on behalf of wild animals shows an analogous logic. It is usually claimed that intervention would have *perverse* effects insofar as it would cause more suffering to the animals living in the wild than the one it aims at preventing or reducing. On occasions, intervening in nature to alleviate animals from natural harms is seen as *futile*. Given the vast amount of suffering that exists in the wild and the multiplicity of natural threats, the impact of such

---

[1] Hirschman (1991).   [2] Ibid., p. 7.

particular actions on animal well-being would be insignificant. Very often, intervention is opposed based on its potential to *jeopardize* other important values, for example, by having a negative impact on the ecosystem's balance or on biodiversity. Thus, the opposition to intervention in nature can be mapped into three different categories of reasons:

(1) *Perversity*: Intervention will have consequences opposite to those intended.
(2) *Futility*: Intervention will have none of the intended consequences whatsoever.
(3) *Jeopardy*: Intervention will threaten other important values.

Nevertheless, Hirschman's taxonomy does not provide us with a complete map of all the objections to intervention. For example, it is often claimed that whether we ought to intervene or not, or whether intervention is merely permissible, depends on the existence of some morally relevant relation. This objection requires an independent category in the taxonomy:

(4) Relationality:
  (a) Intervention is usually not required but merely permissible because we usually do not engage in certain morally relevant relationships with wild animals.
    Or,
  (b) Intervention is usually impermissible because we do engage in certain morally relevant relationships with wild animals.

Another set of objections claims that we should instead prioritize the alleviation of human over nonhuman or, alternatively, to prioritize the suffering of domesticated animals. If that is true, then we have priority reasons not to intervene in nature on behalf of animals living in the wild:

(5) *Priority*: Intervention is not priority.

It could be argued that if this taxonomy aims at being comprehensive, another crucial objection must be included. It is sometimes claimed that wild animal suffering is simply *intractable* as a problem. For example, even if we desired to eradicate wild animals' diseases, we would have no appropriate ways to act on that desire. That is, it is not a claim about the reasons against intervening but a claim about the impossibility to act in accordance with the reasons there are to intervene:

(6) Tractability: Wild animal suffering is intractable.

Table 4.1 *Taxonomy of objections against intervention*

Decisive reasons not to intervene			Sufficient reasons not to intervene
Factual claims	*Normative claims*		
Perversity			Relationality (a)
Futility			
Jeopardy	Priority	Tractability	
Relationality (b)			

In the remainder of this chapter and in the next ones, I will examine the case against intervention and assess its soundness. This amounts to examining the six objections presented above. Some of them are strictly normative positions, while others appeal to facts, and others to a combination of both factual and normative claims, as displayed in Table 4.1.

Given the dissimilarity among them, the response each of these objections merits is substantially different. The route I pursue may be summarized as follows. In the subsequent sections, I assess the first two objections that fall into the original Hirschmanian categories (perversity and futility). In Chapter 5, I assess the jeopardy objection. These objections have in common the claim that we have decisive reasons not to intervene in nature on behalf of wild animals. They succeed if, and only if, our reasons not to intervene in nature are *stronger* than our reasons to intervene. After examining these objections, in Chapter 6, I proceed to discuss the relationality-based objections. Next, in Chapter 7, I examine the objection that improving human or the well-being of domesticated animals has priority over intervening in nature for the sake of nonhuman animals. Finally, in Chapter 8, I discuss the tractability of wild animal suffering.

4.2 The Perversity Objection

Perversity Objection: We have decisive reasons not to intervene in nature because intervention will have consequences opposite to those intended.

The assumption on which this objection relies is that we have very limited knowledge of how complex ecosystems function. Therefore, it is expected that the outcome of intervention would actually be much worse for animals living in the wild than the present state of affairs. Consider, for example, the prevention of predation. If we were to intervene in order to prevent the suffering and death of prey animals, it is claimed, their population levels would increase far beyond the environment's carrying capacity. A boost in population density would then maximize the suffering and death we aimed at preventing by increasing the scarcity of resources and raising the number of deaths by starvation. Therefore, we should not intervene. The adverse expected consequences of intervention give us decisive reasons to oppose it.[3]

In order to tackle this objection properly, it is necessary to distinguish situations when we know and when we do not know what the net consequences of intervention will be. Consider those cases in which the outcome will not be perverse. Imagine some future state of affairs in which wild animal suffering has been reduced to a significant degree due to human intervention in nature. One can plausibly claim that this type of anti-interventionist would find it preferable to the actual state of affairs for animals in the wild. Let us suppose that the interventionist and the anti-interventionist (for perversity reasons) agree about the strength of our reasons to prevent or alleviate the suffering of wild animals. In that case, there would be no room left for further disagreement between them under circumstances of perfect information.

Let us now assume we do not know what the outcome will be and so have to deliberate under epistemic uncertainty. Being in a state of epistemic uncertainty, however, is not equivalent to being certain that the net consequences of intervening will be negative. It is rather that we are *not sure* about the outcome. In such cases, we ought to decide on the reasons given by the expected value of choosing a certain course of action. Thus, the disagreement between the interventionist and the anti-interventionist may be best canvassed as a disagreement about the expected net value of intervention.

a) Status Quo Bias

Maybe we really have reasons to believe that the net consequences of intervention in nature would be negative. As we shall see, it is also possible that opposition to intervention on these grounds merely corresponds to an irrational preference for the preservation of the status quo.

---

[3] This is the same sort of consideration which Jeff McMahan calls the "counterproductivity objection"; see McMahan (2015, p. 279).

Nick Bostrom and Toby Ord offer a "Reversal Test" to help identify instances of status quo bias.[4] I believe that this Reversal Test can also plausibly show that some of the main objections put forward against intervention, such as perversity objections, also suffer from this bias.

Let us now see what the Reversal Test consists in and how it can help us in the assessment of the case against intervention based on perversity reasons.

> *Reversal Test*: when a proposal to change a certain parameter is thought to have bad overall consequences, consider a change to the same parameter in the opposite direction. If this is also thought to have bad overall consequences, then the onus is on those who reach these conclusions to explain why our position cannot be improved by changes to this parameter. If they are unable to do so, then we have reason to suspect that they suffer from a status quo bias.[5]

So

> *Q:* Considering all the possible consequences of intervention in the wild in order to reduce wild animal suffering, will it be better to allow intervention or will it be better to prevent it?

The anti-interventionist would answer that the best state of affairs is one in which intervention is prevented. The test would then proceed by considering a change in the parameter in the opposite direction and asking:

> *Q**: Considering all the possible consequences of intervention in the wild in order to increase wild animal suffering, will it be better to allow intervention or will it be better to prevent it?[6]

Plausibly, the anti-interventionist would now answer that the best state of affairs is also one in which intervention is prevented. Yet, as Bostrom and Ord point out, this is suspicious:

> [I]f a continuous parameter admits of a wide range of possible values, only a tiny subset of which can be local optima, then it is prima facie implausible that the actual value of that parameter should just happen to be one of these rare local optima.[7]

---

[4] Bostrom and Ord (2006). Bostrom and Ord consider objections against genetic cognitive enhancement that appeal the negative consequences it may have – and, thus, an instance of perversity objections. They use the Reversal Test to show how such objections are affected by status quo bias, so that "when the bias is removed, the objections are revealed as extremely implausible" (ibid., p. 658).

[5] Ibid., pp. 664–665.

[6] For simplicity, in subsequent sections, I will refer to an intervention that aims at increasing wild animal suffering as *harmful intervention*, as opposed to *beneficial intervention*, whose aim is to increase wild animal well-being.

[7] Ibid., p. 665.

If that is so, advocates of the status quo need to prove that they are not suffering from an irrational bias. To do so, they will have to provide an alternative, more plausible explanation for their preference for the status quo over other outcomes. The main way in which defenders of the status quo try to meet the burden of proof imposed by the Reversal Test is by appealing to arguments from risk. Hence, it is necessary to examine the main risk-based arguments against intervention and assess the extent to which they pass the Reversal Test.

b) Risk Based on Past Experience

Some people may claim that past human interventions in nature give us decisive reasons to believe that the risk of present or future interventions would be too high. This seems to be what Peter Singer had in mind when he claimed that

> Judging by our past record, any attempt to change ecological systems on a large scale is going to do far more harm than good.[8]

Admittedly, human intervention in nature is often harmful to nonhuman animals. Many animals that live in the wild are relentlessly hunted and sometimes forcefully held in captivity in very stressful conditions in order to satisfy all sorts of human interests, often the most trivial. However, the scope of these considerations is very limited. First, let us assume for the sake of the argument that those harmful interventions had been carried out with the aim of benefiting nonhuman animals, but unfortunately failed to do so. Then, rather than providing us with grounds on which to object to intervening on behalf of wild animals, these considerations would simply recommend caution toward future interventions in nature. Second, those interventions were not carried out to help nonhuman animals, but to benefit humans. Moreover, they were performed out of an utter lack of concern for the interests of nonhuman animals.

Given all this, our past record cannot clearly work as a sound guide or as a good analog for future action since, until now, interventions in nature have been exclusively guided by anthropocentric reasons. An ethical intervention in nature, based on a concern for nonhuman animals' interests, would be substantially different. What interventionists advocate is precisely that we abandon our former aims guiding our intervention in nature. A beneficial intervention in the wild would avoid (at least, in principle) the

---

[8] Singer (2009 [1974], p. 226).

negative consequences for animals that follow from intervening with purely anthropocentric aims.

Thus, by appealing to the risks of intervening, based on our past experience, perversity objections fail to provide a plausible justification for the belief that the actual state of affairs is preferable to other possible outcomes. Therefore, until other, compelling reasons can be provided in its support, we ought to consider the preference for the current state of affairs as suffering from status-quo bias.

c) Risk Based on Epistemic Limitations

Anti-interventionists could still claim that they are not relying on a status quo bias. Instead, they could claim that there are strong reasons to believe that human beings are, as a matter of fact, incapable of acting in ways that benefit animals without thereby harming others. For example, every time humans intervene in order to prevent animals from suffering from a certain disease, this would increase the levels of suffering of other animals who compete for resources with them, or the levels of suffering of their prey. Moreover, in the worse scenarios, intervention could even cause environmental disruption, by dramatically changing whole ecosystems. This would harm not only some particular animals, but all the individuals that inhabit those ecosystems.

This argument, however, would again be misleading. It seems not to be the case that human beings are, in principle, incapable of obtaining sufficient knowledge regarding the possible consequences of their interventions in the wild. Thus, this version of the appeal to perverse consequences can only be an objection against acting on the basis of insufficient information – something that the interventionist would be perfectly willing to accept.

To be sure, we currently have important epistemic limitations regarding the complexity of ecological systems. Because of these epistemic limitations, we should include in our calculus the possibility of many unforeseen harmful consequences. Nonetheless, the further development of ecological sciences will eventually account for this problem.[9] Moreover, facts about

---

[9] In fact, much of the work already carried out in ecology can shed light on this. Furthermore, humans already engage in a similar calculus when intervening in nature in those cases in which their interests are involved. Such interventions used to be carried out, without considering indirect effects they could have, yet they are increasingly performed after a study of the different effects the intervention may have. The same kind of approach, and grounded on similar knowledge, can be applied when it comes to intervening for the sake of nonhuman animals.

wild animal suffering allow us to conclude that a so-called "ecological disruption" is not necessarily bad for nonhuman animals. Rather, the significant change ("disruption") of certain ecological processes may actually be beneficial to animals that live in the wild, considering how bad their lives are in current ecosystems. Certainly, there are ways to significantly change (disrupt) an ecosystem that would be overall harmful to the animals that live there. That would be so, for instance, if it consisted in increasing the number of small animals that inhabit the ecosystem. Yet many other disruptions would be net good for animals whenever they cause less of them to suffer and die. So, once again, disruptive intervention is prescribed only when, given the knowledge available, the net expected outcome would be positive for nonhuman individuals.

Thus, opposition to intervention based on the risks generated by our epistemic limitations does not provide an adequate reason to prefer the status quo over a better state of affairs for animals.

d) Risk of Dystopian Proportions

An anti-interventionist advocate might push the arguments from risk a little further by claiming that it will always remain possible that intervention in the wild leads to unexpected dystopian scenarios. Those scenarios would be bad to such a great extent that we would have especially weighty reasons to be cautious.

If the appeal to dystopia is intended as a perversity objection to intervening in nature, then it must refer to a worst-case scenario for animals in the wild. That is, a situation in which the net outcome of intervening would not only be negative but tremendously negative for these animals.[10] Thus, it constitutes a subclass of the argument from risk based on epistemic limitations previously discussed that stresses the badness of the consequences that intervention might bring about.

Notwithstanding their psychological allure, however, this kind of appeal to dystopian scenarios cannot succeed in vindicating the status quo. The problem is, first, that we may picture these scenarios as following from every possible state of affairs, including the actual world. That is, for any

---

[10] Alternatively, the appeal to dystopia can refer to a worst-case scenario for human beings. By intervening in nature, human well-being, considered as a distinct important value, would be imperiled. Understood in this way, it cannot qualify as an objection from perversity. What this objection assumes is that human well-being has moral priority over nonhuman well-being, so that in cases of conflict, the former ought to be furthered over the latter. I do not believe this sort of objection from priority works either. However, I will discuss this kind of objections in Chapter 7.

dystopian scenario that might follow from any possible state of affairs distinct from the status quo, there is a comparable dystopian scenario that might follow from it. If so, it is false that considerations of this sort give us reasons to preserve things as they stand, instead of trying to improve them. But, second, this is especially clear in the case of animals living in the wild. Even if worse scenarios are always conceivable (e.g., terraforming), given the magnitude of the harms that animals experience in nature, we can safely consider the current situation as already matching the description of a dystopian scenario.

The implication of the previous discussion is that the possibility of perverse consequences cannot provide us, in an unqualified way, with decisive reasons against intervening to benefit wild animals. Awareness of our epistemic limitations gives us indeed reason to be cautious when evaluating the expected outcome of the interventions we may intend to perform. Because the aim of such interventions is to prevent or alleviate the harms experienced by wild animals, they ought to be performed when their expected result is net positive. Conversely, they ought to be avoided when the net expected result is negative.

4.3 The Futility Objection

Futility Objection: We have decisive reasons not to intervene in nature because intervention will have none of the intended consequences whatsoever.

One might think that both futility and perversity arguments draw from the unforeseen consequences of intervention, and that they therefore share the same basic structure. There is, however, a very important distinction to be made between the two types of arguments. While on the perversity objection intervention produces results opposite to the ones intended, arguments from futility rely on the alleged null effects of intervention. That is, rather than rejecting it as counterproductive, it is claimed that intervention will have no effects at all.

Futility arguments may be developed in two distinct ways, all of which stress the human incapacity to make any progress at the improvement of wild animal well-being through intervention. The first one is based on a claim about the fixed structure of nature, upon which human beings would allegedly be powerless to interfere. Call this the *Structural Futility View*. The second one is based on the extent to which prolonging nonhuman animals' lifespan would be futile with regard to increasing their well-being. Call this the *Substantive Futility View*. Each view presupposes different sets of reasons on which to account for the futility of intervening in nature. So, at least in principle, each of them might perform very differently at the reversal test. Therefore, they require a separate assessment.

a) The Structural Futility View

Let us start the examination of this view by putting it through the Reversal Test. As before, we must first ask:

> Q: Considering all the possible consequences *of beneficial intervention*, would it be better to allow intervention or to prevent it?

The futility anti-interventionist may answer this question in two different ways. They may claim that we should be indifferent between refraining from intervening or performing the intervention since doing the latter would be pointless. Alternatively, they may claim that the best state of affairs is one in which intervention is not performed, if only because in this way we would not waste the effort needed to carry out the intervention. Subsequently, given a change in the relevant parameter toward the opposite direction, one ought to ask:

> Q*: Considering all the possible consequences of *harmful intervention*, would it be better to allow intervention or to prevent it?

Plausibly, the futility anti-interventionist would now answer that the best state of affairs is also one in which intervention is prevented.[11] But, if so, this implies that in order to meet the burden of proof required by the reversal test, futility advocates must now provide compelling reasons for considering that nonintervention brings about the best possible state of affairs, or at least one of the best ones.

According to the *Structural Futility View*, any attempt to improve the situation of animals in the wild will ultimately prove hopeless because nature constitutes a highly structured entity, which humans are incapable of modifying. Consider, for example, the predominant reproductive strategy in nature, which consists in producing as many offspring as possible.

---

[11] It can hardly be denied that many *harmful* interventions in nature prove themselves successful. Here past and present experience provides clear evidence of it. But even conceding the possibility that harmful intervention may not significantly affect the well-being of animals (and hence be futile), the costs of implementing such interventions would give futility advocates reasons for opposing them, so their appraisal should be parallel to the one made in the case of beneficial interventions.

Now consider a scenario in which we intervene in order to benefit those animals who reproduce in this way, for example, by preventing them from being affected by a certain disease. Those who endorse this version of the futility objection would say that even the most successful intervention will have but negligibly beneficial consequences since on average only one of these animals per parent will survive. The others will most probably starve to death or be eaten alive by predators before they reach sexual maturity. Therefore, alleviating certain individuals from disease would be a merely cosmetic act. It is futile, supporters of the objection argue, to improve the well-being of these animals, traditionally referred to as *r*-strategists, when we are incapable of eliminating the reproductive strategy they follow. As Chapter 3 shows, this strategy is the fundamental cause of suffering and death in the wild.

This argument might be more clearly formulated as follows:

(1) The basic structures of nature are the fundamental causes of wild animal suffering and death.
(2) Beneficial interventions cannot alter the basic structures of nature.
(3) Therefore, beneficial interventions are futile with regard to alleviating wild animal suffering and death.

Certainly, the argument points to a very important truth: Basic natural processes are the major cause of animal suffering and death in the wild. Such is the case of the reproductive strategy most widely followed by nonhuman animals. This argument, however, suffers from several flaws.

First, its second premise assumes that the basic structures of nature are fixed and act as insurmountable obstacles to any kind of human engineering of nature. Similarly to what happened with perversity arguments, this can only be understood as a claim about human epistemic limitations regarding the manipulation of the basic structures of nature. But so refined, science provides blatant counterexamples to this claim. Scientific development shows that what we previously thought fixed is becoming increasingly manageable. There are no reasons whatsoever to suppose that the current human inadequacy to successfully interfere with natural processes will stay permanent. Thus, futility advocates seem to be begging the question by assuming rather than arguing for the immutability of these natural constraints.[12]

---

[12] Allen Buchanan terms this type of reaction "the Back-Fire View", in his discussion of perversity-type objections to human enhancement. See Buchanan (2011, p.150).

Faced with these considerations, futility advocates may be forced to deflate their position to a claim about present epistemic limitations to successful intervention. But, again, that would make their position practically indistinguishable from that of an informed interventionist. It gives us grounds to oppose specific instances of intervention in light of our ignorance, yet not grounds for opposing intervention, in general. Thus, futility advocates seem to lack compelling reasons for favoring the actual state of affairs over another, possible one in which an epistemically informed intervention took place. Therefore, since futility arguments fail at meeting the burden of proof required by the reversal test, they can be plausibly said to suffer from status quo bias.

In addition, futility arguments seem to suffer from another problem. Even if we were to concede the truth of premise (2), we would still have reasons to dispute the extent to which intervention would be futile. In the human case, we do not certainly believe that it would be futile to intervene, for example, by immunizing populations against a certain disease simply because we lack the means to eradicate the disease altogether, even under conditions of chronic disease and poverty. Or we wouldn't refuse to rescue human populations that have been isolated due to some natural catastrophe simply because of the human incapacity to prevent this type of natural process. There is no way such interventions to save human lives or alleviate their suffering could be considered futile and therefore be justifiably avoided. Certainly, these examples of intervention are not futile for their individual beneficiaries. And there is no other perspective from which to assess the futility of an act beyond that of the individuals affected by its consequences. If the benefits are clear when human beings are the ones positively affected by intervention, then there are no sound reasons to think differently when nonhuman animals are at stake. Futility arguments may, thus, be suffering from a speciesist bias against intervention.

b)   *The Substantive Futility View*

As stated, there are at least two ways in which a futility argument can be developed. The *Structural Futility View* relied on claims about the fixed structure of nature and the alleged powerlessness of humans to significantly modify it. I shall now examine the *Substantive Futility View*. This is a position that relies, instead, on the claim that prolonging the lives of wild animals has no positive effect on their well-being. Given that most animals likely have lives not worth living, shortening a wild animal's lifespan would be good for most of them, insofar as it would deprive them of a life of net suffering.

Again, we shall start by submitting this view to the Reversal Test:

> *Q:* Considering all the possible consequences *of beneficial intervention*, would it be better to allow intervention or to prevent it?

One answer that could be provided is that we ought to be indifferent between intervening and refraining from intervening. Intervening will make the lives of wild animals neither better nor worse. If, in comparison, failing to intervene will be better for no one either, then we have sufficient reasons to pursue either course of action. Another answer that proponents of this view might offer is that we should refrain from intervening. That is what we ought to do, on this view, in those cases in which intervening – which will benefit no animal in the wild – will impose some costs to those who would carry out the intervention. In these circumstances, intervening results in a worse outcome than failing to intervene.

As before, given a change of the relevant parameter in the opposite direction, we ought to ask:

> *Q*:* Considering all the possible consequences of *harmful intervention*, would it be better to allow intervention or to prevent it?

The advocate of a *Substantive Futility View* would now plausibly answer that the best state of affairs is one in which intervention is prevented, insofar as a *harmful* intervention results in an increase in the suffering of nonhuman animals. However, as we shall now see, this position admits a qualification that would allow for an interference typically considered harmful for nonhuman animals, that is, the shortening of their lifespans.

The argument underlying this qualification of the *Substantive Futility View* would go as follows:[13]

(i) The continued existence of a wild animal for any given time span, because of what life in nature involves, never implies a significant increase of their actual or expected net positive well-being.

(ii) Assuming that it does not shorten their lifespans, intervening in nature in ways that allow for the continued existence of those animals cannot significantly increase their actual or expected net positive well-being.

---

[13] I owe this point to Andrew Williams.

(iii) If the only available forms of intervention in nature amount to allowing the continued existence of those animals without shortening their lifespan, then intervention proves futile with regard to the aim of increasing the animals' net positive well-being.[14]

Admittedly, premises (i) and (ii) correctly describe the situation of most nonhuman individuals. The majority of animals that live in the wild have lives not worth living. In some cases, their continued existence is, as a matter of fact, harmful for them. But, contrary to what this view suggests, this does not mean that we cannot benefit animals by acting in ways that save their lives.

Regarding this, first, it could be plausibly claimed that some animals that live in the wild (e.g., large mammals) have lives that are on the whole worth living – even if they are not lives with a high level of well-being. However, these cases are not representative. When we consider the case of most animals (who have lives that are not worth living), we must bear in mind that the actual reason why they have lives in which suffering prevails is that they are affected by harmful factors such as the ones we saw in Chapter 3. But these are also the very factors that cause them to die when they are very young. If those harms were eliminated, they would not die, but then they would not suffer either. Indeed, individuals are not only benefited when their lives are saved, but also when they are spared of some suffering. So, it is not the case that attempting to do so would be futile in the way that this substantive view suggests.

Second, the plausibility of premises (i) and (ii) are mostly dependent on the persistence of the status quo. That is, this scenario only seems inevitable on the currently prevalent noninterventionist paradigm. For example, it might be the case that providing additional food to a starving population infected with a parasitoid would be futile. Doing it would indeed allow for the continued existence of these animals. Since in this case, however, their existence involves being eaten alive from the inside, feeding them would not bring about, on balance, an increase in their net well-being. Nevertheless, and assuming such consequences are indeed expectable, this only makes sense if we fail to intervene to alleviate other causes of suffering – in this case, by failing to deworm the population.

From within an interventionist paradigm, what we should do is to deworm the population *and* provide them with nourishment when needed. That would certainly result in an increase in the well-being of

[14] Perhaps it may even prove perverse, insofar as those interventions allow for the continuation of lives of net negative well-being, which may have already ended otherwise. However, that would transform the objection from futility I am considering into one a perversity objection, already discussed above.

the animals affected. If we lack the means to do both things, then we ought to estimate what would be the best course of action for all the sentient individuals affected and proceed accordingly.[15]

Of course, the futility advocate might respond to this by claiming that our understanding of how such interventionist enterprise might work is currently so limited that any attempt at intervening now would be pointless. Yet this would transform futility arguments into, again, a rather weak claim about present human epistemic limitations to successful intervention in nature. In conclusion, when subjected to scrutiny, the *Substantive Futility View* cannot provide sufficiently strong reasons for preferring the status quo over an alternative state of affairs. Hence, it seems incapable of passing the reversal test as well.

In this chapter I developed a taxonomy of the main objections against intervention in nature on behalf of wild animals. I did this by elaborating on Albert O. Hirschman's three main theses of conservative opposition to social change (perversity, futility, jeopardy) and showed that the negative case against intervention follows an analogous structure. Yet in order to address the full case I added three more categories to Hirschman's taxonomy: relationality, and tractability. I then moved on to assess the cogency of perversity and futility objections to intervention, according to which intervention will either make things worse or will not succeed at making things better for wild animals. I argued that both objections seem to suffer from status quo bias (they fail at the *Reversal Test*) and that once the bias is eliminated, the opponent cannot succeed in providing us with decisive reasons not to intervene in nature. It simply stresses something perfectly accepted by the positive case for intervention. That is, we ought to intervene in nature *only if* the expected outcome is net positive.

---

[15] I am here assuming that the parasitoid infecting these animals is not sentient, and therefore it has no interests that ought to be considered. Otherwise, if the parasitoid were sentient, then one should take into account how their well-being is affected.

CHAPTER 5

Jeopardy

In the previous chapter, I addressed perversity and futility arguments against helping wild animals. Perversity and futility arguments share the assumption that either by bringing about consequences opposite to those expected or by producing no effects at all, intervention attempted at reducing wild animal suffering will fail to do so. This chapter tackles objections of a different kind, namely the Jeopardy Objection:

> *Jeopardy Objection*: We have decisive reasons not to intervene in nature because intervention would threaten (or jeopardize) other important valuable things.

Therefore, the objection does not necessarily deny that intervention will succeed at reducing wild animal suffering.

As in the previous sets of objections, jeopardy advocates do not necessarily disagree, in principle, with interventionists regarding the value of wild animal well-being, even though as a matter of fact most of them do. In order to have jeopardy-derived decisive reasons not to intervene, it is only necessary that the potential costs of our intended intervention outweigh its potential benefits. The costs and benefits, however, ought not to be calculated considering the unique variable of wild animal well-being, these critics would say. If that were the case, we would be back into something similar to the previous perversity and futility considerations. Instead, jeopardy advocates claim, when deliberating whether or not to intervene, wild animal well-being has to be weighed against other values. Since these values are often mutually exclusive, the scenario that intervention would bring about is expected to undermine these other values. Of course, in order for that loss to generate decisive reasons not to intervene, jeopardy advocates will have to show that (i) the status quo is optimal regarding the promotion of those other values and that (ii) we have stronger reasons to promote those values than the reasons we have to promote wild animal well-being.[1] The sort of values typically appealed to are environmental ones.

Jeopardy objections may be developed in several ways, depending on the environmental values they appeal to. The aim of this chapter is to provide an assessment of three main versions of the jeopardy argument against intervention, together commonly known by the generic "environmentalist objections." These are three ways of opposing intervention by means of appealing to the threat that the promotion of wild animal well-being would constitute to environmentalist values. They can be classified into holistic objections, biocentric objections, and the appeal to the natural and to the wilderness.

Again, since each objection has a different way of accounting for the environmental threat posed by intervening in nature, each of them requires a separate assessment.

5.1 Holistic Objections

One way of opposing intervention is by endorsing a form of ethical holism according to which the morally considerable entities are the ecological wholes of which nonhuman animals are a part, such as ecosystems, species, biocenoses, the biosphere, or biodiversity. Individual animals are taken to be either not morally considerable at all or, alternatively, considerable to a much lesser extent. Here, I will focus on two of the most widespread versions of holism in the literature: ecocentrism and the position that defends the preservation of species or biodiversity.

a) Ecocentrism

Ecocentrism rests on Aldo Leopold's famous claim that independently of the harms or benefits caused to its individual constituents, "a thing is right when it tends to preserve the integrity, stability, and beauty of the biotic community. It is wrong when it tends otherwise."[2] This is so because in

---

[1] Disregard for the harms suffered by nonhuman animals in the wild is fairly common among environmental ethicists. See, in particular, Callicott (1980, 1988); Sagoff (1984); Rolston III (1992); Hettinger (1994). For exceptions that celebrate the natural processes that harm animals, while regretting the suffering and death they cause, see Naess (1991); Everett (2001); Raterman (2008).

[2] Leopold (1989 [1949], pp. 224–225).

ethical holism individuals have mere instrumental value,[3] determined by the contribution of their species to the "stability, integrity and beauty" of the so-called "biotic community," which is the ultimately intrinsically valuable entity. Since intervention to promote wild animal well-being is expectably disruptive of the "integrity, stability and beauty" of ecosystems, we have decisive reasons to oppose it.

Note that this is a conditional claim: We ought to oppose intervention if it threatens the preservation of the ecosystem. Of course, ecocentrism does not provide any reasons on which to oppose current and future interventions that prove to be not disruptive to ecosystems (as already discussed with perversity objections). But let us assume, as those who endorse this view do, that intervention in order to alleviate the harms that animals suffer in nature would always *jeopardize* the preservation of a certain ecosystem. The ecocentric objection could thus be refined and specified in the following way:

> We have decisive reasons not to intervene in nature because intervention would threaten (or jeopardize) the preservation of ecosystems.

There are four serious problems with ecocentric holism.

(i) Status Quo Bias

One might first ask if holistic arguments against intervention succeed at the *Reversal Test*. As in the case of the previous objections, given two possible scenarios, one in which a beneficial intervention is carried out and one in which it is not, holists believe that we should favor the latter over the former. A change in the parameter in the opposite direction also leads holism to favor (in principle) the status quo over intervention, or, at least, to favor it conditionally. That will not be the case whenever harmful intervention will be a means to preserve or restore the balance of ecosystems. As a matter of fact, the harmful interventions often performed in nature are based on a holistic rationale. Despite the harm inflicted on the individuals that inhabit the ecosystem, common practices of environmental management consist in this type of intervention. Some examples are the

---

[3] Individual animals have an instrumental value, which is a function of both the value of the species they belong to and its population density. The value of a species is determined by its ecological role. See Callicott (1980, pp. 325–326).

reintroduction of predatory species in an ecosystem where they had been absent or the eradication of non-autochthonous species from an ecosystem, both of which aim at contributing to a new situation of balance.[4]

The aim of these interventions is always restorative of the status quo ante human intervention. We must note, though, that ecosystems are constantly changing. In addition, other ecosystems previous to the present ones existed long before humans appeared. Yet, no interventions are carried out to reintroduce those previous ecosystems. This suggests that ecocentric opposition to intervention has double standards and might be based on an irrational preference for the current state of affairs (in the case of wild areas) or for the state of affairs previous to human presence (in the case of areas already transformed by humans). In order for ecocentrism to make a compelling case against intervention, it would have to be the case that ecocentrism rightly identifies the kind of things that are intrinsically valuable, and that it offers a sound argument regarding what intrinsically valuable entities are to be favored in cases when some can only be promoted at the expense of others. Otherwise, we should consider that the criterion for selecting a certain time as the location of the optimal balance is arbitrary.

(ii) Ecosystems Are Not Like Organisms or Societies

Ecocentrism allocates intrinsic value to the so-called "biotic community," from which the instrumental value of its individual members is to be derived. One of the most salient proponents of ecocentrism, John Baird Callicott, suggests the following two analogies to support this view: [5]

(a) The preservation of an organism's well-being requires the sacrifice of some of its parts, "which cause stress and often pain to various parts of the body and a more rapid turnover in the life cycle of our individual cells."[6] Likewise, the preservation of the "well-being" of the biotic community requires the sacrifice of some of its parts (e.g., the suffering and death of some animals living in the wild).

(b) The preservation of the "interests" of society requires the sacrifice of the interests of some of its parts. Likewise, the preservation of the "interests" of the biotic community requires the sacrifice of the interests of some of its parts (e.g., the interests of some nonhuman animals that live in the wild).

---

[4] For criticisms, see Shelton (2004); Horta (2010d).   [5] Callicott (1980).   [6] Ibid., p. 323.

However, in the case of the organism, it is true that the whole has a well-being of its own whilst it is false that its parts have a well-being. Thus, it is not a case of the well-being of some parts being sacrificed for the well-being of a whole. Therefore, even if we accept the sacrifice of some of our body parts for the sake of the organism, we are not thereby forced to accept that we have reasons to maintain the stability of the biotic community through the sacrifice of the well-being of its members.

In the case of society, it is false that the whole has a well-being of its own that is non-reducible to the well-being of its members. Assuming that there are occasions in which the interests of some members of society have to be sacrificed for the sake of the preservation of society, that will only be the case insofar as the preservation of society is instrumentally valuable for the satisfaction of the interests of other of its members. Therefore, either we assume that this is a false analogy for "biotic communities," or assume that this is a true analogy, so that "biotic communities" have instead instrumental value for the well-being of its members.[7] But certainly, what this holistic view wants to defend is that ecosystems have intrinsic value, independently of how they contribute to the well-being of its members. If that were not the case, ecocentrism would fail to provide reasons with which to object to those interventions informed by research, which might nevertheless threaten ecological wholes.

At any rate, given that the first analogy does not work either, we have no reasons to accept that "biotic communities" have intrinsic value and that we ought to prevent interventions that threaten it. On the contrary, we have reasons to support such interventions based on wild animal well-being. In fact, if consistently adopted, ecocentrism would lead us to highly implausible scenarios regarding the consideration of individual sentient beings, including human beings. This leads us to a further problem.

(iii) Unacceptable Consequences for Humans

If we should prevent the satisfaction of individual interests whenever they may threaten the preservation of the ecological wholes, then we should also prevent human interests from being satisfied when doing so would thwart the "integrity, stability and beauty of the biotic community." For example, by not feeding human beings or not curing them from diseases in underdeveloped areas of the world.

---

[7] As the evidence provided in Chapter 3 suggests, ecosystems do not have instrumental value for the well-being of its members.

Nevertheless, even accepting that human beings represent a major threat to the stability of ecosystems, most people, including the majority of holists, would reject the implication that their interests are to be sacrificed as a means to ecosystem conservation.[8] When the aim of preserving the "biotic community" clashes with the aim of promoting human well-being, most would claim that the latter should be favored over the former. However, when combined with an anthropocentric qualification such as this one, ecocentrism relinquishes its core tenet, namely, that the value of ecosystems is always prevalent when in conflict with the interests of individuals. Given the requirement that moral differences between sentient individuals ought to be established on morally relevant attributes, eco-centrism, so combined with anthropocentrism becomes unacceptable for additional reasons.

(iv) Speciesism

What we have just seen leads to a another problem. This is that ecocentr-ism succumbs to anthropocentric speciesism. In order to avoid the specie-sist charge, it would be necessary to establish a morally relevant difference between humans and nonhumans such that we would have compelling reasons to treat their similar interests differently. However, we have seen already that there is no such morally relevant attribute. This means that the unequal consideration of similar human and nonhuman interests is unjus-tified and that any position that assumes it will also fail to have justificatory power.

In addition, the analogy with the human case and its implausible consequences points to the irrelevance of the preservation of ecosystems in moral deliberation. What is relevant when deciding how we should act is how the interests of individuals might be affected by what happens to them and both human and nonhuman animals have those interests. Thus, it is unjustified to intervene in nature to help human beings in situations of need but to fail to do so in similar circumstances when the beneficiaries are nonhuman animals. Ecocentrism fails to provide a sound justification for opposing to those interventions in nature that pursue the promotion of wild animal well-being.

To be sure, J.B. Callicott has famously attempted to reconstruct Leopold's view in order to avoid such counterintuitive implications, in particular, for the consideration of human interests, arguing that ecological interconnectivity should not be understood in terms of the subordination

---

[8] A salient exception can be found in Linkola (2009).

of the individual to the reality of the whole, but in terms of "accretion" of morally considerable communities structured in concentric circles of "intimacy." Moral obligations would therefore be a function of the level of closeness that we maintain with different communities, so that when in conflict, benefiting the most "intimate" communities would take precedence over benefiting the most distant communities. Thus, for instance, it would not be justified to sacrifice human interests (close community) for the benefit of the biotic community (distant community), but it would be justified to do so when it comes to wild nonhuman animals (distant community).[9]

For some people, this idea has the clear advantage of accounting for basic moral intuitions according to which we should give priority to the interests of those with whom we are involved in "kinship" relationships. However, it could be said that, while it is doubtful whether proximity (geographical, affective, temporal, etc.) is in general a sufficiently robust foundation to account for our moral obligations toward other human beings, it is particularly weakly equipped to account for potential moral obligations toward the nonhuman elements of the natural world, with whom we do not, in principle, maintain close relationships of any kind.[10] Furthermore, if it is true that, from a purely descriptive point of view, moral agents are closer to the human community than to the biotic community, it seems that they are similarly closer to animal communities than to the biotic community. Accordingly, it would not be justified to sacrifice the interests of nonhuman individuals so as to preserve the biotic community. Thus reconstructed, the holistic proposal falls prey of ethical parochialism, simply stating that we should give priority to those to whom we already give priority. In other words, holism becomes a mere reaffirmation of the anthropocentric status quo, moving away once again from its original purpose.

Despite the problems mentioned, holism still has its supporters. The attraction seems to perhaps lie in its alignment with a certain popular ontology according to which "we are all part of a whole" and "all natural phenomena are interconnected." It is true that ethical holism often presupposes other forms of holism, such as ontological holism, the position that there are "wholes" independently of their constituent parts. However, there is a mistake here. It is the case that if we defend ethical holism, we are to some extent committed to ontological holism. However, conversely, to

---

[9] Callicott (1989).
[10] This idea will be fully developed in Chapter 6, dedicated to the relationality objection.

say that "ecological wholes" exist does not imply that they should be morally considered. In other words, it is perfectly compatible to be an ontological holist and to reject ethical holism. For example, one might argue that we are part of an ecological whole, but that it is the parts (or at least certain parts), and not the whole, which are susceptible to moral consideration.

b) Species Holism

A different version of holism would appeal to the intrinsic[11] value of species or biodiversity. Species, some would say, are valuable in themselves, independently of their ecological role or of the impact of their continued existence on the lives of individuals. Insofar as intervention in order to alleviate wild animal suffering might thwart this value (by leading some species to extinction), we should oppose it. The objection can be presented as follows:

> We have decisive reasons not to intervene in nature because intervention would threaten (or jeopardize) the preservation of species diversity.

Despite its popularity, the claim about the intrinsic value of species requires some clarifications.

First, as it was just remarked, if something is non-derivatively valuable, then it is valuable in itself, independently of the benefits or harms that other beings may derive from its existence. This should be distinguished from the idea that what is bad about the extinction of a species is that it is bad for its members. Clearly, this is a mistake since extinction does not affect individuals whatsoever. Individuals (at least, those who are sentient) are not harmed by extinction but only by death (and the process of dying, when it is painful). Moreover, death harms animals individually, and such harms obtain independently of the number of them that belong to a given species. The last individual that dies need not be more harmed by death than the one that died 1,000,000 individuals before them. It is the death of its last individual member that produces the extinction of a species and not the other way around. If extinction is bad, then it cannot be bad in itself in a person-affecting way. That is, it cannot be bad because it is bad for someone.

---

[11] I use "intrinsic value" to refer to telic value, that is, to how something is valuable as an end instead of merely as a means to obtain something else that is valuable as an end.

Second, on this view, species are thus thought to have intrinsic value impersonally.[12] The idea behind this is that the existence of some things can be good or bad even if it is good or bad for no one. Species, some claim, are that kind of thing. When a species becomes extinct, it is argued, there is an irreplaceable loss of value such that the world becomes a worse place than it was before. That is, there is a decrease in the world's overall value. This is what it means that the extinction of a species is bad, even if it is bad for no one. If species can be valuable in this way, then we have impersonal reasons to preserve them.

But, again, this seems to be highly implausible on account of the consequences that embracing such a position has for the consideration of human interests. First, this implication is clearly unacceptable when there are human beings at stake, as not all extinctions seem to be bad.

Consider the case of some extinct non-sentient parasites affecting humans. If every extinction is bad, then the extinction of that parasite must also be bad, despite being good for human populations. Moreover, if the value of species is understood as impersonal, then a state of affairs in which that parasite is not extinct is better than a state of affairs in which it is extinct. If that was the case, then we seem to have reasons to reintroduce the parasite, if it ever became feasible. However, the claim that the parasite should be reintroduced in order to restore the value that was lost with its extinction is hardly plausible. This is primarily because its reintroduction would have a tremendous negative impact on the well-being of human populations. Thus, even if we had reasons to reintroduce the parasite based on the intrinsic value of species, they would be outweighed by the reasons given by human well-being.

Thus, it seems that our value assessments when it comes to species conservation are conditional to their impact on human well-being. This suggests that for most of us, either species are not impersonally valuable – but rather good or bad depending on whether their existence is good or bad for someone – or, alternatively, that their impersonal value provides us with less weighty reasons than those we consider human interests to give us. Given that the interests of a sentient nonhuman animal have no less moral weight than similar human interests, the same considerations should apply when their well-being is at stake.

---

[12] For a distinction between person-affecting values and impersonal values, see also Glover (1977); Parfit (1984, Part IV).

A different route is to claim that species also have a well-being derived from the integrated functioning of their components. However, it is quite difficult to grasp what the well-being of a species would amount to beyond the aggregate well-being of the organisms that compose it. Let us consider the case of *Lynx pardinus*. What exactly is the well-being of the *Lynx Pardinus* species as distinct from the total well-being of its members.[13] Sure, it would be a mistake to infer from the fact that certain constituents of species have their own well-being, that the cluster itself has a well-being of its own. Thus, references to the well-being of a species seem to be, at best, a figurative way of referring to the aggregate well-being of its individual members. But, again, this would be incompatible with holism.

Certain positions could further argue that the *Lynx pardinus* (or any other) species is not a mere collection of individuals, but an entity in itself, which possesses properties not applicable to its individual constituents, such as being in danger of extinction (Nelson 2010). The *Lynx pardinus* species would thus have a well-being of its own or an interest in continued existence over time beyond, and fundamentally distinct from, the well-being (or interests) of its members. There is something right about this idea. On the one hand, it is certain that what is best from the point of view of the preservation of species does not necessarily coincide with what is best from the point of view of individual well-being; it is quite often the opposite. Captive breeding or translocation of individuals, among other conservation measures, plausibly contribute to the preservation of the species at the expense of individual well-being. On the other hand, as we have seen, extinction does not, strictly speaking, affect individuals. What affects individuals (at least those who are sentient) is death or the process of dying when accompanied by suffering. However, considering that the extinction of species can be bad from an impersonal point of view does not support the thesis that species have a well-being of their own or an interest in continued existence over time.

Thus, due to its implausible axiology and its unacceptable consequences for the consideration of human interests, holism seems incapable of providing compelling reasons to oppose intervention for the benefit of nonhuman animals.

---

[13] Particularly, considering behavioral and physiological indicators typically used in the overall assessment of well-being, among them, food levels, shelter, health, and appropriate behavior of individuals (Botreau et al. 2007, Fraser 2008).

Finally, and on a different note, many interventions simply do not threaten whatever values holism pursues. For instance, species holism lacks grounds on which to oppose those interventions that do not bring about species extinction. For its part, ecocentrism cannot successfully object to aiding animals within constantly interfered ecosystems, such as urban, or peri-urban ones. Moreover, on certain hybrid views, even though considerations about non-sentient entities might limit intervention to help wild animals, they might not pose a significant threat to the claim that we should in general help wild animals in need.[14]

5.2   Biocentric Objections

Biocentrism is the position according to which the set of morally considerable beings consists in all forms of life. Thus, it includes within the realm of moral consideration not only sentient animals but also all other non-sentient living organisms such as plants, fungi, or bacteria. Biocentric views typically claim that every living thing has a "good of its own" that should be respected by not being interfered with.[15]

The biocentrist argument against harming living beings may be specified in the following way:

(1)   Every living thing has a well-being of its own.
(2)   Every entity with a well-being of its own has intrinsic value.
(3)   Respecting the intrinsic value of a living thing amounts to refraining from harming it.
(4)   Therefore, we should not harm living things.

Applied to intervention, the biocentrist argument might be formulated as follows:

(5)   Every intervention that harms living things disrespects the intrinsic value of those living things.
(6)   Intervention in nature harms living things.
(7)   We should prevent disrespect for the intrinsic value of living things.
(8)   Therefore, intervention in nature should be prevented.

Thus, the biocentrist objection could then be refined to read:

---

[14] See Cunha, Luciano C. (2015) If natural entities have intrinsic value, should we then abstain from helping animals who are victims of natural processes? *Relations: Beyond anthropocentrism*, v. 3, n. 1, 51–63.
[15] See, for instance, Schweitzer (1973 [1923]); Taylor (1981, 1983, 1986); Agar (1997); Sterba (2011).

We have decisive reasons not to intervene in nature because intervention would threaten (or jeopardize) the lives of living organisms.

One might now ask how the biocentrist objection performs at the *Reversal Test*. If being alive is the criterion for moral consideration, it follows that both beneficial and harmful interventions for sentient beings should be prevented insofar as they can be harmful to other living things. But, of course, one would then have to ask in what way the status quo constitutes a better scenario regarding the "well-being" of all forms of life than the one following after intervention. Suppose we accept that not only sentient beings have a well-being. If so, the status quo is in fact a threat to the "well-being" of a great number of living organisms, whether they are sentient or not. There is a permanent conflict of interests between different forms of life in nature: diseased animals devoured by bacteria, fungi nourishing from plants, plants eaten by herbivores, and predators feeding from prey. Thus, abstaining from interfering does not preserve the "well-being" of all forms of life. Instead, it enforces the naturally arbitrary way by which the "well-being" of some living organisms is favored over the well-being of others. So, it seems that there are no compelling reasons based on the intrinsic value of all forms of life for preferring the status quo over other scenarios, namely the one in which beneficial intervention takes place.

In addition, there would still be other reasons why it would fail to provide a successful objection to intervention. We will examine them in the following section.

a) *Biocentrism's Axiology*

The first problem biocentrism has to face is related to its allocation of value. Consider premise (1) of the biocentrist argument. The idea is that if an entity is alive, then it has a well-being of its own. That is, things can go well or badly for it. However, this claim is based on a mistaken assumption, namely, the equivalence between the fulfillment of biological needs and well-being. A plausible conception of well-being requires an affective condition that makes it possible for an event to be experienced as good or bad. Even though for some living beings satisfying their biological needs (or failing to do so) amounts to an increase (or decrease) in their well-being, this is clearly not the case for every living thing that exists. Only sentient beings satisfy that requirement. Insofar as they can have positive and negative experiences of what happens to them, things can go well or badly for sentient beings. What happens to them can increase or detract from their well-being, and hence they can be benefited or harmed by events that concern them. Thus, even though being alive is a necessary condition for having a well-being – insofar as being alive is, at least contingently, a prerequisite for having experiences – it is not a sufficient condition.

It is important to dwell on this point since references to the alleged "well-being" of plants are still quite widespread. What are we talking about exactly when we claim that sunlight and water are "good" for a plant? In this respect, Alasdair Cochrane's distinction between prudential and perfectionist value can be of help. According to Cochrane, while prudential value concerns how life goes for individuals themselves, perfectionist value concerns what makes something a good member of its kind. When we say, for instance, that oil is "good" for a bicycle, we are invoking a perfectionist value rather than a prudential value. Surely, lubricating a bicycle will allow it to go smoother and thereby make it a better member of its kind. Yet the bicycle itself does not have an interest in being lubricated, nor it is good for it. The same applies to sunlight or water being "good" for a plant. An adequate amount of sunlight and water will prevent the plant from decaying. It will flourish, in a biological sense, thereby becoming a good member of its kind. Yet, it is not prudentially good for the plant itself to receive sunlight or water. Just like bikes, plants have no well-being of their own and, therefore, no interests. They cannot be harmed or benefited by what happens to them.[16]

The implication for biocentrism is that grounds for the claim that all living things have intrinsic value cannot be the fact that they have a well-being of their own. Biocentrism cannot invoke the prudential value of living things since they have none. The correspondent obligation of respect is therefore unwarranted. There is, of course, still room for an argument that would ground respect for living things on their perfectionist value. Notice, however, that in order to succeed, that argument would have to offer reasons for pursuing perfectionist values over prudential values. Needless to say, assuming the bike analogy stands, those reasons would be rather weak.

b)   Conflicts of Interests

The second problem biocentrism faces is related to its consequences when conflicts of *interests* take place. If all living things have intrinsic value, then

---

[16] Cochrane (2018: 17). But see also Cochrane (2012).

we should take the *interests* of all living things into account, including beings such as bacteria and other non-sentient organisms. Leaving aside the previous problem regarding the attribution of interests to non-sentient entities, this leads us to highly implausible scenarios in which we lack criteria to make comparative assessments between sentient and non-sentient interests. For example, there is no way of solving the clash between the interest in not suffering of a squirrel infected by a parasitic disease and the *interests* of the bacteria themselves in being alive. Of course, to many of us the claim that the *interests* of a bacteria should prevail over the interests of a squirrel not to suffer and eventually die in a slow and painful way seems unreasonable. Perhaps, the example becomes clearer if we substitute the squirrel with a dog. Or, alternatively, if we substitute the dog with a human baby.

c) Speciesism

Biocentrist authors typically avoid this implication by establishing certain conditions under which it would be justified to favor human interests against the interests of nonhuman living entities.[17] For example, when basic interests are at stake, such as in the case of the baby infected by a parasitic disease. This is very intuitive indeed. When well-being is at stake, we believe that we should act in ways that alleviate the suffering of individuals even if that implies terminating the lives of bacteria. Since bacteria have no experience of what happens to them, they cannot be harmed by death in any significant moral way. On the contrary, sentient beings such as human babies can. So, even conceding that non-sentient entities are recipients of value, when preserving that value implies detracting sentient beings from well-being, we have compelling reasons to prioritize the interests of sentient beings.

Nevertheless, there are no nonarbitrary reasons on which to ground this human exceptionalism (see Chapters 1 and 2). There is no sound way to justify favoring human interests against the "interests" of non-sentient living entities and failing to do the same regarding similar nonhuman interests. To deny this implication is to imbue biocentrism with anthropocentric speciesism. Thus, either biocentrism is consistent and all living things have a similar intrinsic value that should be equally considered, or biocentrism gives priority to the interests of sentient beings against the interests of non-sentient living entities, independently of the species

[17] Taylor (1986).

they belong to. The first option (consistent biocentrism) turns biocentrism into a highly implausible theory. The second one amounts to a combination of biocentrism with a view that grants consideration to sentient beings. Since speciesism is unjustified, we would have reasons for intervening on behalf of nonhuman animals. As it is apparent, the many problems that follow from embracing biocentrism make it a highly defective moral position. Ultimately, biocentrism fails to provide a compelling case against beneficial interventions in nature.

5.3   The Appeal to the "Natural"

One of the most widespread objections against intervention takes the form of an appeal to the natural or, alternatively, to the (natural) wilderness.[18] Appeals to nature are usually classified as a fallacy, that is, as the ungrounded inference that something is good because it is natural. Yet, it would be uncharitable to claim that the case against intervention in nature by appeal to the natural or to the wilderness could be reduced to a mere appeal to nature. In what follows, I will thus reconstruct two more sophisticated versions of the objection and assess their cogency.

a)   The "Natural" as the Result of Evolution

The first objection to intervention made by an appeal to the natural could be reconstructed as follows:

> We have decisive reasons not to intervene in nature because intervention would threaten (or jeopardize) the preservation of "the natural," where "the natural" stands for the natural processes by which evolution operates.

The objection relies on the axiological assumption that the result of evolution is good. Insofar as interfering with natural processes amounts to interfering with what is valuable, we should abstain from interfering with nature.

One can immediately foresee how appeals to the natural perform at the *Reversal Test*. If natural processes are valuable, any interference with nature detracts from what is valuable. Thus, a change in the relevant parameter in the opposite direction, such that a harmful intervention (instead of a beneficial one) is performed, would make no difference in this view regarding the reasons to oppose it. Both interventions would jeopardize

[18] Godfrey-Smith (1979); Katz (1996); Elliot (1997).

the natural (understood as the result of evolution) to the exact same extent. As any interference that might threaten it is to be avoided, both would be objectionable.

The argument may seem appealing. However, even though it may be the case that the status quo is optimal regarding the natural (except to the extent to which previous human intervention has disrupted evolutionary processes), it is not clear that what is optimal in terms of the natural coincides with what is optimal in terms of the good.

One way this identification of the good and the natural could be defended would be to assume a teleological understanding of evolutionary processes, that is, the idea according to which evolution resembles a "master engineer" and operates in a rather purposeful way. This would make of the status quo a fraction of a balanced system perfectly organized by some sort of naturally intelligent design. However, this clashes with the view of natural history we have since Darwin. Since nature has no purpose, it cannot have a good purpose either.

Alternatively, we may think that natural selection tends to select traits that are favorable to organisms, including sentient animals. This view, however, is incorrect. Darwin himself disputed this idyllic view of nature when he wrote: "What a book a Devil's chaplain might write on the clumsy, wasteful, blundering, low and horridly cruel works of nature!"[19]

The words chosen by Darwin pinpoint the exact features that describe evolutionary processes. This is so because natural selection selects for reproductive fitness (or for traits promoting reproductive fitness) alone, without regard for the costs on individuals. As a matter of fact, by selecting for reproductive fitness, natural selection consistently selects *against* individual well-being. Consider the results of the main reproductive strategy followed in nature, which increases the transmission of genetic information from one generation to another through the maximization of the number of offspring. It results in lives of net suffering followed by death for most of the individuals that come into existence. Thus, the successful transmission of genes (reproductive fitness) rather than being good for individuals is in most cases actually inversely proportional to the maximization of well-being.

This can be seen more clearly if we imagine a Malthusian nightmare in which the human population on Earth has reached the maximum planet's carrying capacity. Assuming that human populations cannot extend beyond the planet, humans would have then reached their peak

[19] Darwin (1856, p. 94).

reproductive fitness (probably at great costs to members of other species). By the time population reaches its peak, human well-being would also be reaching its bottom, with perhaps most humans living lives that are not worth living.

In sum, the status resulting from the history of natural selection is not at the optimal state of affairs for individuals in terms of what is good for them. If that is so, then "natural" becomes a description of "the way in which things happen to be as a result of the processes by which evolution operates." In that sense, appeals to the natural fail to provide us with moral reasons to prefer the status quo over other states of affairs, namely, those in which well-being is increased through human intervention.

b)   The "Natural" as Natural Wilderness

Of course, one might still claim that even though evolution is suboptimal in terms of well-being, the natural should be preserved regardless, since it contains a value of a different kind. But clearly, that argumentative move would call for a different argument, that is, an argument that would show that (a) the natural possesses valuable properties not grounded on being the result of natural selection and (b) those properties provide us with stronger reasons than the reasons given by the value of well-being.

A second objection to intervention based on an appeal to the natural could be reconstructed as follows:

> We have decisive reasons[20] not to intervene in nature because intervention would jeopardize the natural, where the "natural" stands for natural wilderness, that is, the state of being unmodified by the human hand.

Again, faced with the *reversal test*, those who endorse this objection would answer negatively to both types of intervention (beneficial and harmful), insofar as each interference would presuppose a disruptive process from which an irreplaceable loss of a valuable property would follow – its wilderness. Of course, proponents of this view would then have to provide a sound argument on which to base their opposition to

---

[20] Elliot (1997). Elliot does not state that wilderness gives us decisive reasons to oppose intervention, but merely sufficient ones. Nevertheless, even though Elliot concedes that his argument does not aim at establishing (b), I believe it is important to assess the extent to which it does not succeed at establishing (a) either. This is of course independent of whether the property in question provides us with decisive or sufficient reasons to oppose intervention. So my assessment is immune to that potential objection.

intervention that allowed them to meet the burden of proof imposed by the *Reversal Test*, thereby avoiding the charge of status quo bias.

The argument could then go along the following lines, as presented by Robert Elliot:[21] The value of objects is explained to a significant extent in terms of the processes that brought them into existence. Since nature is not replaceable without a disruption of its history, intervention necessarily implies a loss of value. More clearly,

(1) The value of nature depends, at least partially, on its continuity with its genesis (i.e., depends on its wilderness).
(2) Intervention in nature disrupts the continuity of nature with its genesis.
(3) Therefore, intervention in nature disrupts, at least partially, nature's value.
(4) We should safeguard nature's value.
(5) Therefore, intervention in nature should be avoided.

Elliot justifies premise (1) by relying on an analogy between faking art and faking nature.[22] He claims that in the same way as a painting loses a significant part of its value once we realize we had a false belief about its origin (a perfect forgery), a natural area loses a determinant part of its value once we realize that it has been modified by human hands (as implied by intervention).

Before going into assessing Elliot's argument, it is important to clear the ground regarding a more general challenge that appeals to wilderness are usually confronted with. As it has been extensively pointed out, "wilderness" is a problematic concept on both empirical and philosophical grounds.[23] On the empirical side, it needs to be acknowledged that there is hardly any place on Earth today that has not been in some way interfered with by human action, though it is certainly true that if "wilderness" is to be understood as an "endpoint of a spectrum of human choices, actions and historical trajectories,"[24] the objection loses much of its force. Yet, a lot would still remain to be said regarding many "natural environments" that presently stand as the result of human action. These include urban, semi-urban, and agricultural ecosystems, as well as many mountains and forests, where, as a matter of fact, much of the death and suffering that intervention seeks to reduce occur. Such a position could not object to helping animals in such circumstances.

---

[21] Ibid. [22] For a similar analogy, see Dworkin (1993, pp. 73–75).
[23] Keeling (2008) for a critical overview. [24] Keeling (2008, p. 506).

Regarding the philosophical side, it has been argued from within environmental ethics that the concept of "wilderness" relies on an untenable human–nature dualism, according to which the products of human activity and those of nature belong to entirely different, and mutually exclusive, ontological spheres.[25] This belief, however, presupposes a pre-Darwinian conception of human beings as not being part of the same evolutionary (natural) processes as the rest of living entities. The only continuity there is, the argument goes, is natural history, and hardly anything (not even human action) falls outside its scope.[26] This core idea is captured by Aldo Leopold's famous passage: "Wilderness is the raw material out of which man hammered the artefact called civilisation."[27] There is no sharp discontinuity between human activity and the natural entities and processes through which and out of which humans carry out such activity. In that sense, human activity is no less separate from nature than the construction of a beehive or the crafting of tools by chimpanzees.

Despite the wide support for this view, I believe it would be misleading to ignore the ambiguity of the terms being employed. As John Stuart Mill noted centuries ago, debates "[o]n Nature" contain a fatal ambiguity since "[t]he word "nature" has two principal meanings: [I]t either denotes the entire system of things, with the aggregates of all their properties, or it denotes things as they would be, apart from human intervention."[28] Clearly, while environmentalist detractors of the idea of wilderness use "nature" or "natural" to refer broadly to everything that exists, including human action – Mill's first -, Eliot and other defenders of the idea of wilderness use "nature" or "natural" to refer specifically to that which exists or occurs independently of human agency – Mill's second sense. Thus, they are simply talking past each other. To be sure, detractors of the idea of wilderness would likely insist that the narrow sense of "nature" and the nature/culture dualism associated with it is still problematic, not the least because it is incompatible with ecological holism, according to which human activity is "one" with all other evolutionary phenomena.[29] This does not follow, however, since ecological holism does not entail ontological monism. But, at the end of the day, it seems that the value of wilderness (or lack thereof) should not depend on whether human activity is a part of nature or not.

[25] See Nelson and Callicott (Eds.) (1998, 2008). For other criticisms based on wilderness alleged ethnocentric, androcentric, and phallocentric nature (among others), see Nelson (2007) for an overview.
[26] Callicott (1998).   [27] Leopold (1989 [1949]).   [28] Mill (1902).
[29] Callicott and Nelson (1998, 2008).

Now, back to Elliot's argument from analogy between fake art and fake nature, it seems that the alleged analogs are different in the relevant aspects for comparison purposes. In the case of works of art, it is clear how there is some discontinuity between the production of the fake painting and the genesis of the original one, that is, the process by which it came to be out of the intentional states of its creator. No matter how perfectly forged the painting is, there is no causal link between the object and the intentional states of the original author. Contrariwise, in the case of nature, there is no original creative activity to which to appeal.

First, natural processes are not the expression of the intentional states of a creator and certainly there is no purpose in them (except figuratively and, even then, none other beyond the maximization of reproductive fitness, as we have seen before). Since the most plausibly relevant aspect of continuity is its correspondence between the author's mental states (its genesis) and the final creation, this *genetic* aspect is completely absent when it comes to the natural world.

Second, and most importantly, the genesis of a painting does not negatively affect other aspects of the painting's value. Whereas in the case of nature, given the predominance of natural disvalue, its genesis does so necessarily. This is precisely the reason why we should aim at modifying it. Interestingly enough, Elliot introduces a second analogy that correctly traces this idea, despite not being aimed at that goal. Elliot considers a scenario in which a beautiful artifact is offered as a gift to someone who then realizes that it has been carved out of someone's bone, who was specifically killed for that purpose. He claims that the object would immediately lose a significant part of its value. Regrettably for him, though, this example does not help his case. In fact, if anything, the example shows exactly the opposite: The value of the object depends greatly (if not entirely) on its impact on the well-being of others. If the genesis of an object caused a negative impact on the well-being of a human individual, then the object cannot be as valuable as some might initially think it to be. Likewise, once we realize that natural beauty is carved out of the misery and death of nonhuman animals that live in the wild, the value of the natural wilderness fades away.

Third, this understanding of nature has very extreme "hands-off" implications. According to this view, no human interference in the environment, even those carried out to restore or preserve natural entities, can be justified.[30]

---

[30] Godfrey-Smith (1979); O'Neill, Holland and Light (2008).

In conclusion, jeopardy objections based on any version of the appeal to the natural do not succeed at objecting to intervention.

Some might be inclined to say that the present analysis fails to be thorough insofar as it leaves out pluralist approaches to the moral considerability of environmental entities.[31] I will now briefly tackle this issue. The pluralist view, though diverse, is premised on the belief that an adequate moral theory must be able to capture the "dynamism" and "complexity" of life and the moral phenomena associated with it. It follows that questions of moral considerability (on which the case for and against intervention greatly relies) cannot be based on a single criterion or principle so that the reasons for considering different types of entities will vary. For example, there are certain properties of a psychological nature, such as rationality and autonomy, whose possession makes an individual morally considerable. This does not mean that moral considerability should be restricted to those entities that meet such conditions. Individuals with more rudimentary cognitive abilities, by virtue of having their own well-being derived from sentience, are equally considerable. Other forms of non-sentient life must also be taken into account in attaining their natural achievements, and the same applies to "ecological wholes" and natural processes. That is, there are a variety of moral reasons for considering different entities, and they are all compatible with each other. Depending on the particular situation, some reasons or others are called for.

There are clear difficulties with such a view. While it is true that, in general, moral decision-making and, in particular, moral deliberation about environmental matters are complex and confusing, greatly due to our epistemic limitations, it does not seem to follow that our best theoretical efforts should mimic the confusion and pre-theoretical complexity. The fact that there is a plurality of possible considerations to accept that P, does not imply that our best reasons for accepting that P are plural. Plausibly, if there is one thing that theory should aspire to, it is precisely to resolve conflicts between plural and contradictory beliefs and to identify nonarbitrary reasons to prefer one course of action over another. It is not clear, therefore, to what extent pluralism offers a response to conflict resolution that arises when considering that nonhuman entities, even nonliving ones, should be similarly morally considerable, which can escape the accusation of arbitrariness and inconsistency in moral action.

It is true that, in general, pluralist views minimize the importance of consistency, claiming that it is the price to pay to guarantee inclusivity in

---

[31] See, for instance, Stone (1987), Wenz (1988), Hargrove (1985), Cheney (1989).

the moral sphere and caution in decision-making.[32] There are several problems with this idea though. First, theoretical inclusiveness is not *in itself* good. What we want from a theory is not that it is inclusive simpliciter but that it is relevantly inclusive. That is, it is based on nonarbitrary reasons to include certain entities and to exclude others. It would be implausible to think that a theory that includes living beings and cobblestones within the scope of moral considerability is better than a theory that only includes living beings, on the basis that the former is more inclusive than the latter. Second, being aware of risk and uncertainty in moral decision-making does not imply a commitment to pluralism. Careful moral reasoning is sufficient. The cogency of pluralistic approaches to intervention will ultimately depend on whether pluralism is an appropriate approach to morality more generally. Of course, this is not the place to assess the merits of pluralism as a general theory. Yet, there are already a number of problems that cast serious doubts on the robustness of the proposal.

In this chapter, I assessed the cogency of jeopardy objections to intervention, according to which intervention to reduce wild animal suffering should be prevented, on the basis that it threatens other (more) important values. These are the preservation of ecological wholes (holism), the preservation of other living non-sentient entities (biocentrism), and the preservation of what may be called "the natural" and "the wilderness." I showed each of these individual approaches fails. Even if we suppose nature has all these grounds of value combined, that does not help the non-interventionist case unless, that is, one is ready to embrace anthropocentrism or bite the bullet or unreasonable conclusions regarding human beings. Of course, one could say another plurality of values must be appealed to, but then one would have to show which are these different values and provide an argument against intervention. Until that argument is provided, I conclude that jeopardy objections cannot soundly oppose intervention in nature for the sake of wild animals.

[32] Marieta (1993).

CHAPTER 6

Relationality

The previous chapters examined the first set of objections against intervention in nature, namely, those based on considerations of *perversity*, *futility*, and *jeopardy*. It concluded that none of these objections succeeds in defending the claim that we have *decisive* reasons to oppose intervention. The following chapters provide an assessment of the second set of objections against intervention. This chapter addresses the challenges to intervention laid out first, by Clare Palmer and then by Sue Donaldson and Will Kymlicka. It groups and labels both positions in what we may call *relationality* objections.

Relationality Objection:

(a) Intervention is usually not required but merely permissible because we usually do not engage in certain morally relevant relationships with wild animals.

Or,

(b) Intervention is usually impermissible because we do engage in certain morally relevant relationships with wild animals.

6.1 Palmer's Contextual Approach

Clare Palmer is one of the few authors who directly address the problem of animal suffering in nature and the moral obligations it may generate. She does so from the contextual account of the moral consideration of nonhuman animals, which she has extensively developed.[1] Palmer claims that we are not usually required to assist wild animals. However, we may be permitted to do so. Her thesis relies on two premises, which we may collectively call

[1] Palmer (2010, 2013, 2015).

The Relevant Entanglement Argument:

(i) We are morally required to assist others in need *if, and only if,* we have a prior *morally relevant entanglement* with them.

(ii) Usually, there is no such *morally relevant entanglement* between human beings and wild animals.

The argument can be illustrated with a comparison Palmer draws between two real-life cases. Consider the situation of 114 horses left starving to death by their owners. If it was in our power to do something to alleviate their suffering, ought we to do it? Would it be wrong to let them suffer and die if we could otherwise help them? The usual response to this case is that failing to assist these animals would be wrong. But then, Palmer asks, if this is the case, does it imply that we should assist other animals in a situation of need? What about the animals living in the wild? They experience systematic suffering and have premature deaths. As Palmer exemplifies, every year there is a massive drowning of wildebeest during their migration from Tanzania to Kenya. Were it feasible, should we then intervene and prevent them from such harms? Both cases involve animal suffering and death. Let us assume for the sake of the argument that human assistance in both cases (horses and wildebeests) would generate the same outcomes regarding the total amount of suffering relieved. It seems that if we just take into consideration the interests of the animals involved, then we should make a similar decision in both situations.

Notwithstanding the similarities between the two cases, however, Palmer claims that we tend to believe that while there is an obligation to help the horses in the first case, we are not required to intervene on behalf of the wildebeest in the second one. What goes on in the wild, most people think, is not our moral business. Palmer believes that the difference in our intuitive moral responses to these cases is indeed justified. The "laissez-faire intuition," as she calls it, adequately captures our (usual) lack of positive moral obligations toward animals in the wild:

> *The laissez-faire intuition*: While we have obligations to assist and care for domesticated animals, we have no such obligations toward animals in the wild.[2]

Palmer's default position is, thus, that there is no general moral obligation to help others in need. Instead, we merely have special obligations of assistance toward those individuals with whom we have *morally relevant*

---

[2] Palmer (2010, p. 63).

entanglements. It is the existence of such entanglements that generates obligations of assistance. Since human beings and wild animals (e.g., wildebeest) usually do not maintain these morally relevant relationships, helping them is merely permitted, as opposed to morally required. And we may decide to exercise that permission by refraining from assisting them.

In Palmer's view,

> *Prior morally-relevant entanglement* refers to any causal relation between an individual's particular situation of exposure to a harm (which generates the need of aid) and past human action.

Domesticated animals – such as the horses in the example – are a paradigmatic instance of this. As she points out,

> [...] where humans have deliberately created relations of dependent vulnerability with animals (especially where this involves prior harms, such as wild capture), special obligations to care for these animals, and to assist them, are also created.[3]

That is, we are required to prevent or alleviate the suffering of domesticated animals because we deliberately put them in a situation of vulnerability and dependence. If the argument is sound, it allows Palmer to establish a morally relevant difference between domesticated animals and those living in the wild, in spite of their having similar morally relevant capacities (equal capacity to suffer and enjoy their lives).

Palmer draws on a human analog for support: the case of parents' special obligations toward their own children. Even though all children have similar morally relevant capacities, she claims, we only have special obligations to assist our own, since we are in some way responsible for putting them in a situation of vulnerability, by having brought them into existence. Likewise, despite their similar levels of suffering, we have only special obligations toward the animals we have deliberately made dependent and vulnerable through domestication. In sum, we should assist domesticated animals (but not those living in the wild) not because their well-being is threatened by some harmful event, but because we are responsible for making them vulnerable to that threat.

Palmer's view, then, is not that we have decisive reasons not to intervene to help animals, but that we have enough or sufficient reason not to do so. Thus, her argument succeeds just if it cannot be shown that our reasons to intervene are stronger than our reasons not to do so.

---

[3] Palmer (2015, p. 207).

Consider, again, the analogy that Palmer establishes between special obligations toward domesticated animals and those toward one's own children. The point of the analogy was to show that, just as we have special obligations toward our own children in virtue of having caused their coming into existence, we have special obligations to domesticated animals (and yet, not to wild animals) in virtue of having deliberately put them in a situation of dependence and vulnerability.

However, this analogy does not prove as much as Palmer intends. Conceding that parents have special obligations toward their own children, it does not follow that they do not have reasons to assist other children in need. It might simply be that their reasons to assist their own children are stronger than those to assist other people's children. In fact, most people would consider it impermissible not to assist a child, let's say, about to be crushed by a rock, if we could otherwise help them, on the grounds that we are not responsible for making them vulnerable to that situation. If this is so, then even if it were right that our reasons to assist domesticated animals were stronger than our reasons to assist wild animals, it would still be unjustified to fail to assist animals in the wild.

Thus, this argument from analogy cannot ground Palmer's strong view that obligations to assist individuals in need only arise from prior morally relevant entanglements. As a matter of fact, Palmer seems to be aware of this alternative to her view when elsewhere she claims,

> There might be a different version of this view – that requirements to assist do exist in such cases but that they are much weaker where there's no prior entanglement; however, I don't have space to develop such a view here.[4]

However, the latter would not merely be a different version of Palmer's view but a completely different one. And this weak relational thesis is, indeed, the one that most plausibly follows from Palmer's arguments. However, it does not claim intervention to aid animals in the wild is not required. Only her stronger thesis does. But such a thesis has very counter-intuitive implications. Immediate worries arise in its application to the human case, as Palmer herself acknowledges. If our reasons to assist other individuals are generated by a causal link between present suffering and previous human action, there seems to be no requirement to help distant human beings in need due to natural causes. If we have not made these human beings vulnerable to that harm (what is generally true of harms

---

[4] Palmer (2013, p. 29).

caused by natural events), we have no obligation to assist them. Palmer attempts to avoid this implication by further specifying her argument:

> [T]he entanglements of human societies, in particular the social and struc-
> tural connections between virtually all people, connections that benefit
> some while causing suffering to others, provide a basis for human obliga-
> tions to assist other humans [. . .].[5]

One plausible way of understanding Palmer's answer to what generates these *special obligations* of assistance among human beings is that special obligations of assistance are generated by causal relations.

According to this, all harms that human beings suffer are directly or indirectly caused by the social and structural connections among human beings that benefit some while causing suffering to others. This view seems, however, highly implausible. First, it is not true of all harms. There are clear cases of harms that humans suffer that cannot be traced back to human action. Paradigm examples of these are diseases, as well as natural catastrophes such as earthquakes, tsunamis, floods, droughts, etc. If Palmer is right, we would have no obligation to help those humans in need suffering from these and similar natural events. Thus, it would be false that her account provides a basis for human obligations to assist other humans in need.

One might say against this that there is a relevant difference between both cases since the humans who suffer the harms belong to the same network of relevant connections as those humans whose actions are partly responsible for the harms, whereas wild animals do not. However, that reply would be misguided in two different ways. First, if an individual is harmed by an action or event, then that individual immediately enters into the relevant network of connections with an agent. One may say that insofar as an individual is in need, that is, there is something that they lack in order to avoid being harmed, they are engaged in a relationship with moral agents with respect to the meeting of their needs. No other morally significant relationships have to obtain between the parties for moral obligations of assistance to arise. To accept this when the victims are human and deny it when the victims are nonhuman would be an instance of speciesism.

Second, let us suppose that the relevant connections that allegedly hold among human beings, and which ground special obligations among them, are not causal in the sense that they can be directly or indirectly traced

---

[5] Palmer (2015, p. 207).

back to human action but, instead, refer to certain other kinds of relations, which hold between individual human beings, such as

> mutually recognized communication, the ability of humans to justify them-
> selves to others, reciprocity in economic relations, mutual cooperation, the
> joint organization of political and other institutions, membership of political
> communities, the sense of a political "world order," and membership in
> families.[6]

If that were the case, then special obligations to assist would not arise toward all human beings either. This is because there are human beings who fail to engage in the aforementioned relations. It is clearly the case that some human individuals, by virtue of their functional diversity (especially in those cases in which such mental diversity is very significant) or other circumstances, do not engage into "mutual communication." Nor do they reciprocate or enter into any political, economic, or familial relations. Hence, we would also lack any obligations to assist them, even if it were in our power to do so. Thus, unless Palmer accepts that we lack the obligation to assist human beings that do not satisfy these conditions, her view does not provide a sound basis for excluding nonhuman animals from the scope of those obligations (e.g., wild animals).

Moreover, the moral relevance of these entanglements in establishing obligations of assistance can be questioned altogether. Assuming that it was feasible to help those individuals without jeopardizing similarly weighty interests, we ought to provide them with the assistance they need. This is so because the cause of the harm that individuals suffer does not affect the weight of their interests in not being harmed. For example, the interest in not suffering from a leg injury inflicted by another human is, all things being equal, as strong as the interest in not suffering from a similar injury caused by the fall of a tree. Thus, if human interests in avoiding suffering and in living their lives are relevant independently of other considerations, and if those interests are equally weighty independently of who or what frustrates them, taking them into account requires two different courses of action. First, it requires that we refrain from harming these individuals. Second, it requires that we prevent them from being harmed by other events or that we alleviate unavoidable harms they endure (e.g., by preventing their deaths or by reducing their suffering). Thus, it would be unjustified not to act according to either way of accounting for other

---

[6] Palmer (2010, p. 121).

individuals' interests, whenever it is in our power to do so. This can be clearly observed in the following scenario.

Suppose that you are presented with these choices:

(i) Press button A: All human beings are immunized against all lethal forms of cancer.

(ii) Press button B: Only those human beings with whom we are engaged in "morally-relevant entanglements" are so immunized.

(iii) Press no button.

Palmer's view would imply that we are morally required to press either B or A – thus, we may permissibly choose not to press A. This is because our special obligations of assistance are completely satisfied by pressing button B.[7] However, most people would find this odd. Assume that the costs of pressing either button are the same. Also, more individuals are benefited when A is pressed than when B is. So, it seems that any view that does not require an agent to benefit others even when that comes at no cost, not even to the agent themselves, is hardly acceptable.

Of course, in real-world cases, helping always bears a cost for the agent or for others. Yet this scenario does not aim to show that we should not take costs into account when deciding whether we should help others. If this is correct, it shows that we are required to help others even if we are not relevantly entangled with them in the ways specified by Palmer.

Now, suppose that it were feasible, and had similarly low costs, to help a wild animal population, say, by rescuing it from a flood or by vaccinating it against an extremely painful disease. Failing to do so would constitute a similar disregard of their interests. Such as in the human case, what generates an obligation to help these nonhuman individuals is the importance of their well-being, the extent to which it is threatened by some event and our possibility to intervene in order to help them without causing a greater harm.

---

[7] Notice that this is not even one of those cases in which, according to Palmer, pressing button A, even if not required, would constitute a display of virtuous dispositions. This is because this is not a situation involving an immediate encounter with an individual in need with whom we do not have morally relevant entanglements (see the *Squirrel* case in Palmer 2010, pp. 148–150). Moreover, if immediate encounters with individuals in need elicit certain dispositions to act, then it seems that such dispositions would be elicited more generally in a larger set of contexts, depending on the extent to which we put ourselves in a position to have immediate encounters with individuals in need. This becomes particularly clear when considering the central case of wildebeest drowning during migration examined by Palmer (2010). Contrary to Palmer, by choosing to place themselves in a position of bystander exposure to the suffering of wildebeest (as many tourists do), and by not intervening, moral agents would also be failing to display the morally adequate dispositions.

Some may argue that helping wild animals would then be morally required only when doing so has low costs. It would not be required, however, when the costs are non-negligible. Consequentialists will disagree, of course, but others could also challenge this view. For some non-consequentialists, aiding others at some non-negligible cost is supererogatory *when* the situation in which others are is not catastrophic. However, when failure to intervene will cause a truly enormous amount of harm, and the costs of intervention are affordable, even non-consequentialists will agree we are required to intervene. At least, non-consequentialist which simultaneously accept the existence of positive obligations, excluding only some libertarians.

Thus, when deciding whether we should help wild animals, the magnitude of the harms they suffer is usually underestimated. As Chapter 3 extensively argues, it is highly probable that the lives of the majority of wild animals contain much more suffering than well-being, which, on aggregate, makes suffering largely predominant over well-being in nature.

These facts are crucial since once we have questioned the relevance of the kind of entanglements Palmer specifies, the most important factors to take into account when deciding whether or not to assist others have to do with how much they can be benefited and at what cost. Given the magnitude of wild animal suffering, usually the costs of intervening in order to help them will be significantly smaller than the benefit they may receive. Additionally, in the case of wild animals, the cost they must bear when their suffering is not relieved is very high. Thus, we have strong reasons to conclude that we ought to assist them. This can be accepted not only on a consequentialist view but also on many non-consequentialist perspectives.

6.2 Donaldson and Kymlicka's Sovereignty Argument

Sue Donaldson and Will Kymlicka claim that interventions to benefit wild animals should respect the relations of sovereignty that ought to be established between human political communities and the so-called "wild animal communities."[8] On this view, though all nonhuman animals equally have a set of negative rights, only those that enter into some relations with human beings enjoy positive rights. Even though, in some sense, Palmer's and Donaldson and Kymlicka's accounts are both relational in nature, Donaldson and Kymlicka's relational approach is considerably different. On this view, it is not the case that we do not maintain

---

[8] Donaldson and Kymlcika (2011a).

morally relevant relationships with wild animals. Yet different political relationships determine different moral obligations. While some animals enter
into relationships of co-citizenship with human beings (by virtue of fully or
partly belonging to human communities), the morally relevant relationship
between human beings and wild animals is one of sovereignty. As they say,

> Our suggestion is that the relationship is best captured by ideas of sover-
> eignty – that is, we should view wild animals as forming organized com-
> munities, competent in general to address the challenges they face and to
> look after their own needs and interests, who typically neither need nor
> want their lives to be managed or governed by humans.[9]

This, as Donaldson and Kymlicka remark, will lead to a conclusion that is
substantially different from the one to which Palmer arrives. Their argument[10] might be synthesized as follows:

(i)   Contrary to Palmer, it is not the case that domesticated animals are
      dependent on X, where X is any means to satisfy their needs, and
      wild animals are not. This is because both depend on X to satisfy
      their needs.
(ii)   Regarding whether we are considering domesticated or wild ani-
      mals, X stands for different things.
(iii)   We have a positive duty to ensure that all animals obtain X.
(iv)   For domesticated animals, X stands for some "relationship to
      human beings." Positive *specific* duties are generated.
(v)   For wild animals, X stands for some "relationship with the natural
      environment." Positive *nonspecific* duties are generated.

     Thus, contrary to Palmer,

(vi)   We have a positive (nonspecific) duty to respect the dependency of
      wild animals on their natural environment.

In order to illustrate the point of this objection, consider again Palmer's
analogy with parenthood. From the fact that we may have specific duties
toward our own children (e.g., to provide food, shelter, and medical care),
it does not follow that we lack any positive duties toward other children in
need, even though our duties toward other children may differ from the
duties we have toward our own in that they are nonspecific duties. That is,
they are nonspecific in the sense that they are duties to ensure *whatever*
enables other children's basic needs to be met. Since, according to

---

[9] Donaldson and Kymlicka (2011b, p. 9)   [10] See Donaldson and Kymlicka (2011, pp. 207–208).

Donaldson and Kymlicka, wild animals depend on their natural environment to meet their needs, we have a duty to ensure that their environment provides for the satisfaction of their needs.

Subsequently, Donaldson and Kymlicka deploy the second part of their argument.

Assuming that

(vii) Wild animal populations are sufficiently competent for successfully engage into self-government – that is, they are sufficiently able to exercise all the necessary functions to thrive without external intervention.

Then,

(viii) The best way to respect the dependency of wild animals on their natural environment is to establish relations of *sovereignty* with wild animal communities.

Remember that according to Palmer we lack compelling reasons to benefit animals in the wild, either by providing them with some good or by preventing them from a natural harm. Wild animal interests do not provide us with decisive reasons to intervene on their behalf. On the account we are considering, on the other hand, the assertion of sovereignty rights acknowledges the moral relevance of wild animal interests. First, these rights impose restrictions on human interference with the so-called "wild animal communities." But, crucially, respect for these rights requires intervention whenever "altering nature's course [is necessary] in order to prevent catastrophe" (e.g., devastating illness). Thus, the appeal to the sovereignty of wild animals, as understood by Donaldson and Kymlicka, conflicts with Palmer's thesis that even if intervention is permitted, it is not required.

Even if the Donaldson–Kymlicka view may be too optimistic about how beneficial establishing these relations of sovereignty can be for wild animals (as I will argue below), it makes two important claims that are relevant for the assessment of Palmer's view:

(a) We are morally required to ensure that nonhuman animals obtain whatever it is that they are dependent on in order to meet their basic needs.

And,

(b) In complying with that requirement, "letting nature be" need not always be a better course of action than intervention in nature. Thus, a positive duty to intervene can arise.

Now, one can agree with Donaldson and Kymlicka in their general criticism to Palmer's account and yet question (i) their diagnosis of wild animal competence to self-govern and (ii) the adequacy of the sovereignty rights response to the moral relevance of wild animal interests. Such disagreement, though, would seem to be essentially based on empirical grounds.

As Chapter 3 shows, nature, far from it being a source of well-being for wild animals, is rather a source of intense misery. Data from population dynamics tells us that due to the reproductive strategy favored by the majority of wild animals, suffering plausibly predominates over well-being in nature. The fact that a population thrives does not imply that its members do flourish, but rather that the overwhelming majority of them may have short lives, full of suffering.

This renders the claim that wild animal populations are sufficiently competent to self-govern extremely implausible. Wild animal populations, as some have claimed, are better described as "failed states."[11] In this sense, it is false that, as Donaldson and Kymlicka think, the best way to respect the dependency of wild animals on their natural environment is to establish relations of sovereignty with wild animal communities.[12] The satisfaction of wild animals' interests does not depend, as the authors believe, on the preservation of their natural environments since the preservation of their natural environments amounts to continuous suffering and death for most animals that come into existence. Thus, if we have a duty to ensure that their environment provides the satisfaction of their needs, sovereignty rights of the sort Donaldson and Kymlicka have in mind are not the solution. On the contrary, the adequate way of complying with the requirement to attend to wild animals' needs is some form of what I shall call *environmental enhancement*.

> *Environmental enhancement*: any modification of natural environmental conditions that produces a net positive effect on the well-being of sentient individuals.

---

[11] Mannino (2015); Horta (2013); Cochrane (2013).

[12] Alternatively, one might say that intervention would not in any relevant sense violate the potential sovereignty of animals in nature. This may be because wild animals are not sovereign but rather equal members of mixed human–animal communities (Cochrane, 2018). In that case, intervening in nature would be a duty of domestic justice. Or, it may be that intervention in nature to help animals is analogous to a situation of humanitarian intervention regardless of species membership. In that case, while wild animals may form sovereign communities, intervening on their behalf would be a duty of international justice on Donaldson and Kymlicka's view. Either way, intervention follows.

The argument can be presented as follows. If,

(i) We are morally required to ensure that nonhuman animals obtain whatever it is that they are dependent on in order to meet their basic needs

and

(ii) Animals' natural environment is such that often their basic needs are insufficiently satisfied, or not at all,

Then,

(iii) We are morally required to enhance animals' natural environment in order to ensure the adequate satisfaction of their needs.

The general conclusion is, thus, that even though Donaldson and Kymlicka's assessment of Palmer's view correctly identifies serious problems with the account, it remains too optimistic regarding the net effect of animals' natural environment on their well-being. This leads to a view that resembles much more a "let nature be" position than one that challenges nature as a "flat moral landscape,"[13] as was initially intended by the authors.[14] Nevertheless, as I have argued, once we acknowledge the magnitude of wild animal suffering, it may still be possible to make room within their theory for the satisfaction of wild animal interests, via the prescription of *environmental enhancement*.[15]

Some might object to this, of course, by claiming that environmental enhancement should be prevented due to its potential perverse or futile effects. Nevertheless, as Donaldson and Kymlicka themselves acknowledge, "[...] we can't hide behind the fallibility argument for non-intervention

---

[13] Donaldson and Kymlicka (2011a, p. 6).

[14] Some might say that Donaldson and Kymlicka's position would be better accommodated under the jeopardy set of objections to intervention. That would be so insofar as intervening on behalf of wild animals would threaten the value of wild animals' sovereignty. Nevertheless, I believe that would be a mistake since, according to Donaldson and Kymlicka, sovereignty is understood as instrumentally valuable for the promotion of wild animal well-being. On another interpretation, Donaldson and Kymlicka's position would be better described as a perversity objection, insofar as intervening on behalf of animals would be, all things considered, worse for them. This is because even in those cases in which intervention would be successful in terms of alleviation of suffering, that would negatively affect the autonomy of these nonhuman individuals. Moreover, this would be so in such a way that the harm inflicted to animal *autonomy* would not be compensated by the reduction in suffering. However, even the authors admit that this overall net-negative assessment only holds under the assumption that wild animal communities are sufficiently competent for self-government. As shown in Chapter 3, however, they are not so. Thus, understood as a perversity objection, Donaldson and Kymlicka's view fails in its own terms to provide us with decisive reasons against intervening.

[15] As a duty of international justice, one might add. See footnote 12.

insofar as our impact is already pervasive and unavoidable."[16] Having addressed these objections regarding the more general opposition to positive intervention in Chapter 4, I will assume here that no compelling reasons of this kind can be provided to oppose environmental enhancement either.

There is one specific way to oppose environmental enhancement by appealing to perversity, which is through an appeal to considerations of *flourishing*.[17] As a matter of fact, this seems to be a quite widespread position among the general public used to resist intervention in nature, even though it is not as prevalent in the philosophical debate.[18] Applied to environmental enhancement, the flourishing objection might go along the following lines. Environmental enhancement should be prevented insofar as it undermines the flourishing of wild animals, where "flourishing" stands for acting in accordance with the kind of being a creature *is* (or according to a creature's own *nature*). In other words,

> *Flourishing*: A being flourishes if, and only if, they act in accordance with their own set of characteristic traits and capacities, which have evolved due to natural processes.

However, as prominent theorists in the field have pointed out, there is no equivalence between the result of natural processes and an individual's *flourishing*.[19] Moreover, "flourishing," understood here in evolutionary terms, stands for a mere description of what dispositions sentient individuals happen to have at the present point in evolution, which, as previously explained, in itself, carries no moral weight. Thus, it cannot help build up a moral case against environmental enhancement.[20]

In addition, attaching axiological or moral relevance to this conception of "flourishing" leads to very counterintuitive scenarios. Suppose that an individual who is a member of type X acts according to dispositions y and

---

[16] Donaldson and Kymlicka (2011a, p. 164).

[17] The appeal to flourishing could indeed be extended to a more general opposition to intervention based on considerations of perversity. For the sake of simplicity in the exposition, I am addressing it here.

[18] A salient exception can be found in Everett (2001).   [19] See Hadley (2006); Nussbaum (2006).

[20] Appeals to flourishing might be alternatively understood in a way that allows them to resist this objection. It might be said that what is morally relevant is not that such and such traits are the result of natural processes, but rather that what is relevant is that individuals live in certain ways, which can only be ensured if some natural processes are preserved. Nevertheless, as thoroughly discussed in previous chapters (particularly in Chapters 1 and 2), what is morally relevant is instead the extent to which an event increases a sentient individuals' well-being or detracts from it. Thus, the preservation of natural processes is conditional to its impact on individual well-being. Yet, as we have seen in Chapter 3, natural processes are precisely what causes the low levels of wild animal well-being.

z, where acting on y and z is a means to successfully carrying out the life cycle of members of type X. Once we have already established that x is acting on such dispositions, and once we have accepted a definition of flourishing according to which to flourish is to act on such dispositions, it would be redundant to ask whether x is flourishing. If to flourish *is* to act in accordance with the set of naturally evolved characteristic traits and capacities that allow the successful life cycle of a certain type, then if a being acts in accordance with those traits and capacities, that being is flourishing. But if to flourish is to act in accordance with the result of evolutionary processes, then flourishing does not seem to be something valuable.

A simple example laid out by Peter Singer might help to illustrate this point:

> Suppose that a man who has the means to acquire and maintain a harem of women who proceed to bear him dozens of children, is as flourishing as anyone can be. So, for that matter, are the women fortunate enough to be selected for the pampered and secure life child-bearing that membership of a strong, wealthy man's harem involves. If we deny that such men and women are flourishing, we are introducing evaluations that need to be explained.[21]

An alternative explanation of what is going on with our intuitions regarding this case is that while there might be a certain respect in which these men and women are flourishing, there is another important respect in which they are not – not in terms of well-being. But, of course, there is no reference to individual well-being on the considered conception of a being's "flourishing" as *acting in accordance with their own set of characteristic traits and capacities, which have evolved due to natural processes*.

First, one may consider that flourishing solely consists of individual well-being. In that case, we would be using the term in a completely different way:

> *Flourishing*: A being flourishes to the extent to which they have a net positive level of well-being.

If, more plausibly, we understand flourishing in this different sense, then it is false that environmental enhancement undermines the flourishing of wild animals. Consider food availability, an important limiting factor of wild animal populations. Despite the scarcity of resources, animals come into existence in great numbers, most of them typically dying of starvation

---

[21] Singer (2002).

shortly after birth. The rest that does survive, for the most part, suffer from malnutrition and experience a prolonged and harsh death, characterized by the progressive loss of bodily functions and by extreme distress. Clearly, these animals cannot be said to be flourishing in any sense that matters since they have lives of net negative suffering. Thus, environmental enhancement, far from being detrimental to animals, would actually ensure that the necessary conditions for their flourishing, understood only in terms of well-being, would be met.

Second, one might still disagree with this by claiming that, even if welfare is a necessary condition for flourishing, it is not a sufficient one. The best definition of "flourishing" would be:

> *Flourishing"*: A being flourishes if, and only if, (i) they act in accordance with the set of natural evolved characteristic traits and (ii) they have a net positive level of well-being.

But, again, as previously explained, there are no compelling reasons on which to believe that acting on her "naturally evolved traits" in any way positively contributes, by itself, to an individual's flourishing. Indeed, acting on many such traits is clearly harmful to the nonhuman individuals whose flourishing we are assessing (e.g., boundless procreation[22]). It is certainly implausible to claim that all naturally evolved traits are equally desirable in terms of individual flourishing. So, a proponent of this view would have to provide a distinction between naturally evolved traits that are relevant for flourishing and those traits that are not. Plausibly enough, the relevance of such traits should be appraised by their impact on individual well-being. But, of course, if the relevant set of naturally evolved traits is fixed by how it affects individual well-being, then condition (i) of acting in accordance with such set of traits turns out to be superfluous. Thus, *Flourishing"* should be rejected as an adequate conception of flourishing.

In sum, what I claim should be Donaldson and Kymlicka's commitment to environmental enhancement cannot be objected to by appealing

---

[22] Some might say that procreation is not a good example of how a naturally evolved trait or disposition can impinge one one's own flourishing, insofar as it seems to impinge on the flourishing of one's offspring instead. Yet, data suggests that traits that increase reproduction are favored by natural selection, even if they reduce individual maintenance, often, at the expense of individual survival. This is particularly true of female individuals. See, for instance, Cruz-Flores et al. (2021); Culina et al. (2019); Dobson and Jouventin (2010); Koivula et al. (2003); Proaktor et al. (2008). By way of curiosity, in humans, the costs of reproduction are also correlated with a decrease in health and longevity (Jasienska 2020, Jasienska et al. 2017) and an increase of the risk of cognitive decline (Ziomkiewicz et al. 2019).

to flourishing considerations. If "flourishing" is defined as an individual's behavior being in accordance with a set of naturally evolved traits, then this objection begs the question against environmental enhancement by assuming, rather than proving, the moral relevance of natural processes and their outcomes. If, on the other hand, "flourishing" is relative to how well off an individual is, then the objection lacks any grounds on which to oppose environmental enhancement since the vast majority of wild animals are prevented from flourishing, primarily, by natural processes. Finally, on a possible pluralist conception of "flourishing," reference to behavior in accordance with naturally evolved traits turns out to be superfluous. It is thus incapable of providing new grounds on which to oppose environmental enhancement.

An additional remark regarding Donaldson and Kymlicka's stance on the flourishing objection to intervention on behalf of wild animals is still necessary. Though in *Zoopolis*, the authors reject the objection, they also claim that

> Our approach [...] is a theory of sovereignty which recognizes that the flourishing of individual wild animals cannot be separated from the flourishing of communities, and which reframes the rights of wild animals in terms of fair interaction between communities.[23]

That is, the flourishing of individual animals (y) must be understood as a *function* of the flourishing of wild animal communities (x). Thus, the flourishing of individual animals will vary according to whatever value the flourishing of wild animal *communities* takes on, such that $y = y(x)$.

Now, I believe this section has already shown why this cannot be the case. Individual flourishing cannot be defined in terms of an animal *community*'s flourishing since a *community*'s thriving does not imply that its individual members do flourish. On the contrary (as we have seen in Chapter 3), the flourishing of the *community* implies that most of its members have premature deaths and plausibly lead lives of net suffering. Since it is implausible to sustain that, despite that, individuals are flourishing, the equation should be rejected.

Moreover, the equation should be rejected for another reason, which has to do with the adequacy of the term "community" to describe the interactions of nonhuman animals living in natural environments. In its common usage, "community" (c) stands for a certain unified group of individuals, living in a particular area and cooperating in some way for the

---

[23] Donaldson and Kymlicka (2011a, p. 167).

satisfaction of common interests of a certain kind. We can call this the *political* sense of community. In ecology, nonetheless, "community" (c') refers to a group of interacting species living in the same location, unified by a shared environment and a network of influence of each species over others[24] (including predation, competition, mutualism, commensalism, and parasitism). We can call this the *ecological* sense of community. While the overwhelming majority of interactions between animals living in the wild can be rightly described as an instance of c', it would be misleading to describe it as an instance of c. As Chapter 3 shows, wild animal interactions are best characterized as intraspecific hostile competition for resources and interspecific aggression of various kinds. Usually, the ambiguity between c and c' remains unnoticed, and it is suggested that since wild animals are communities c, then they know what is best for them and they should therefore be left alone. Yet "wild animal community" in this sense misdescribes the relations among wild animals. The term "wild animal community" (c) has a null extension. Nothing is a wild animal community in this sense. And if so, then every declarative sentence that includes it is false.[25] Thus, the sentence "The flourishing of individual wild animals is a function of wild animal communities (c)" is also false. Therefore, it cannot provide us with any reason against environmental enhancement, in particular, or against any other intervention in nature on behalf of wild animals, more generally. Moreover, given the persistent ambiguity of "community," this term should be abandoned altogether.

Someone might press this point by saying that it implies that, for instance, a herd or pack made up of members of a social species would not qualify as a community, which seems implausible. However, it seems that the burden of proof is on the side of those who believe that a pack would qualify as a community in the relevant sense. They need to clarify what sense of "community" they have in mind and show that it qualifies as a community for the purposes of what's relevant for Donaldson and Kymlicka's view. It seems, though, that Donaldson and Kymlicka do *not* consider that a "community" of elephants is a community in the strong sense; that is, it is not susceptible to be a subject of a sovereign state. Even if there may be social relations between nonhuman animals – call this a community in a weak sense – those are not the sort of relations that are susceptible to being considered a community in Donaldson and Kymlicka's

---

[24] Horta (2013).
[25] For a discussion of empty terms in moral discourse and the corresponding truth value of the declarative sentences that contain them, see, for instance, Hom and May (2013, 2018).

sense. What they have in mind is rather the relationships between several populations of different species, interacting in the same ecosystem, that is, a community in an ecological sense. Therefore, a herd, a pack, or a mixed-species feeding flock of birds would not qualify as such.

In this chapter, I examined what can be labeled as relationality objections to intervention in nature. In the literature, these have been most importantly addressed by Clare Palmer and by Sue Donaldson and Will Kymlicka. I began by reconstructing Palmer's argument against the existence of a requirement to assist wild animals in the absence of prior morally relevant entanglements with them. I argued against Parlmer's relational objections to intervention in the wild. I also presented Donaldson and Kymlicka's challenge to Palmer and offered a strong case for pressing Donaldson and Kymlicka's account forward in a way that implies that much more pervasive interventions in nature – what I called *environmental enhancement* – may be required. Finally, I addressed some objections to this claim and concluded that appeals to relationality do not constitute sound objections to intervention, especially in light of the magnitude of the harms experienced by wild animals.

CHAPTER 7

Priority

In previous chapters, I challenged perversity, futility, jeopardy, and relational arguments against intervention. In this chapter, I examine another set of arguments against the conclusion that intervening in nature to help animals is what we have most reason to do.

> *Priority Objection*: When confronted with the choice between intervening in nature on behalf of wild animals and benefiting human beings, the latter has priority over the former.

A cogent priority objection to intervention on behalf of wild animals will have to

(i)   Endorse the empirical claim about the widespread presence of suffering in nature (see Chapter 3);

(ii)   Acknowledge the overall benefits of intervention in terms of nonhuman well-being, assuming intervention is feasible;[1]
and,

(iii) Offer compelling reasons for it to be the case that intervening on behalf of wild animals is *not a priority*; hence it is not what we have most reason to do.

It is possible to find three main strategies for (iii) in the literature. Even though they do not explicitly address the case of animals in the wild, there is no reason why we should not understand the scope of such considerations as including wild animals as well.

---

[1] Some might say these two conditions are not necessary in order for a priority objection to obtain. For example, someone might endorse the priority thesis, while being skeptic about the magnitude of wild animal suffering. Alternatively, someone might be skeptic about the overall benefits of intervention (e.g., by accepting some form of futility argument) and nevertheless defend that improving human well-being has priority over intervening on behalf of wild animals. However, for the reasons exposed in previous chapters (mostly, Chapters 3 and 4), those would be very fragile versions of the priority objection. I shall therefore focus on the strongest case against intervention in nature based on priority considerations, which satisfies both of these conditions. At any rate, if my arguments are sound, they will apply to the weak and strong versions of the objection equally.

One way in which benefiting animals in the wild may be morally more important would be if we assumed some egalitarian or prioritarian view.[2] As shown in Chapter 3, these animals have very low levels of well-being (in fact, we could say they have very high levels of net-negative well-being). Arguably, providing them with some benefit would bring about more value than the alternatives because that is what would contribute the most to reduce inequality, or because they are worse off.

Thus, one of the main strategies consists precisely in excluding nonhuman animals from the scope of distributive principles altogether, such as those of priority and equality. Call this *the Exclusion Approach*. This strategy has been followed first and foremost by Jeff McMahan.[3] The other consists in accepting that nonhuman animals lie within the scope of principles of equality or priority yet diminishing the importance of their interests for the purposes of distribution. If the argument is sound, what nonhuman animals are owed is significantly reduced. Call this *the Deflation Approach*. This strategy has been famously pursued by Peter Vallentyne[4] though it was first defended by McMahan.[5]

Finally, there is the view that benefitting nonhuman animals would not bring about more value, given, for instance, a perfectionist axiology. In this case, one need not assume any egalitarian or prioritarian view. This strategy can be found in Parfit[6] as a way to avoid the Repugnant Conclusion, even though the case of nonhuman lives is only very marginally addressed. Throughout the chapter, I will refer to it as *the Perfectionist Approach*.

7.1 The Exclusion Approach

The Exclusion Approach: Sentient individuals below certain cognitive capacities are excluded from the scope of distributive principles, such as equality and priority.

---

[2] Even though these views are very diverse, the arguments put forward throughout the chapter apply both to telic and deontic versions of egalitarianism and prioritarianism. For a distinction between telic and deontic egalitarianism, see Parfit (1995). Additionally, it must be noted that the egalitarian views I am addressing consider that both equality and well-being matter.

[3] McMahan (1996) restricts the Exclusion Approach to equality principles, even though for argumentative purposes it is possible to extend it to priority principles as well. Given the situation of wild animals, if intervention or nonintervention follows from the egalitarian view, it must also follow from the prioritarian view (Section 7.1).

[4] Vallentyne (2005).

[5] McMahan (1996) assumes the Deflation Approach when discussing what he calls "non comparative distributive principles," such as prioritarian views.

[6] Parfit (most notably 2004 [1986] but also 1984).

As previously mentioned, this is a strategy pursued by Jeff McMahan, according to which there are some properties whose possession "makes an individual one's moral equal and thus brings him or her within the sphere of justice."[7] These properties are psychological in nature, identified in the Kantian tradition with those "necessary for moral agency: rationality and autonomy."[8] Thus, sentient beings who lack such complex cognitive capacities are excluded from the *sphere of justice* and hence from the scope of principles of equality and priority.[9]

This strategy can be seen as an instance of a wider moral outlook – the one Richard Arneson calls the Rational Agency Capacities Account[10] – which privileges beings that exhibit the capacities associated with the rational agency. According to Arneson,

> A rational agent can identify available courses of action she might take, discern reasons for and against the options, weigh and assess the reasons she discerns, deliberate and make choices, carry out the action chosen, and do all this not simply for a single decision problem at a time but with respect to long-term plans of action and projects she might undertake. A rational agent can identify reasons that have a bearing on what to do, and this ability to detect reasons includes an ability to understand and appreciate distinctively moral reasons involving the due consideration and concern that each of us owes to others.[11]

On this account, there is a subset of moral considerations that only apply to our treatment of other rational agents and apply to all of them to the same extent. The fact that an individual is a rational agent makes their interests matter in a special way. It is not just that their interests are considered to be more important so that our reasons against frustrating them are stronger than against frustrating similarly weighty interests of nonrational agents. On this account, different principles apply when considering the interests of rational agents. Considerations of equality and priority are valid in their case, while they are not in the case of sentient individuals who are not rational agents. If distributive principles should be

---

[7] McMahan (1996, p. 30).   [8] Ibid., p. 31.

[9] Note that even if nonhuman animals are excluded from these principles, characterized as principles of justice, we may still have other reasons to benefit them, given by non-justice principles. However, I will not pursue this line of argument here..

[10] Arneson (1999, 2014).

[11] Arneson (2014, pp. 34–35). One might further wonder what exactly is the connection between reason or recognition and the importance of equality or priority. Even though Arneson does not explicitly provide an answer to that question, one might hypothesize that there is an implicit link between distributive justice and the possibility of social cooperation. Those who are unable to contribute to cooperation do not have a valid claim to be recipients of distributive goods.

conceived in this way so as to apply only to rational agents, then we have no equality or priority reasons to benefit nonhuman animals.

Thus, applied to the case of wild animals, the argument could be reconstructed as follows:

(i)   Distributive principles (equality or priority) belong to the subset of moral considerations that only apply to beings with p.
(ii) Wild animals do not exemplify p.
(iii) Therefore, distributive principles do not apply to wild animals.
(iv) Hence, we lack equality and priority reasons to intervene on behalf of wild animals.

Now, as some of its proponents sometimes acknowledge, there are several complications with this view.[12] First, complex cognitive capacities (*p*) come in degrees. Consider, for instance, the capacities involved in rational agency. Some rational agents are clearly better off than others in terms of, for example, identifying the relevant reason-giving facts in balancing reasons in an unbiased way or in conforming their actions to the balance of reasons. Thus, there are two options here:[13]

(i)   Equality and priority reasons apply in varying degrees of strength such that the degree to which they apply to an individual is directly related to the degree to which they possess p.

    Or,

(ii) There is a threshold in the scale of p such that equality and priority reasons uniformly apply to all individuals above it, and to none of those below it.

Opting for (i), however, effectively makes the Exclusion Approach collapse with the Deflation Approach, which I will examine in the following section. Thus, for the time being, I will focus exclusively on the threshold hypothesis. As stated, this is the claim that there is a threshold in the scale

---

[12] McMahan (2002, pp. 249–251, 2008); Arneson (1999, 2014).
[13] I will assess the simplest options advanced in the literature, even though the same conclusions would follow for other, more complex views, such as (a) a gradual scale below a threshold and then uniform status; (b) no status below a threshold and then a gradual scale; (c) several thresholds; and (d) a gradual scale above and below the threshold with varying degrees of incline, so that status varies very significantly depending on the capacities of individuals until a certain point is reached and varies only a little depending on those capacities from then on. At any rate, all of these variations are prone to the same objections. For a detailed analysis of the idea of moral status, see Horta (2017b).

of cognitive capacities such that equality and priority reasons apply equally to all individuals above it, and to none of those below it.

On this view, then, complex cognitive capacities (e.g., rational agency) may be a kind of range property.[14] That is, just like all the points within a circle can be counted as equally inside the circle, regardless of their proximity to the center, there is some threshold in the scale of cognitive capacities such that all beings above it can be considered equals for moral purposes, even if, as a matter of fact, they differ among them with respect to those capacities. All individuals below the threshold are excluded from the application of distributive principles (equality and priority). Plausibly, the cognitive capacities of most nonhuman animals would fall below the threshold so that they would not qualify for inclusion within the scope of equality or priority. Hence, we would have no equality or priority reasons to intervene in nature for their sake.

One problem with this approach is that it is not easy to justify positioning the cutoff point at any particular location. This must be so whether we conceive the threshold as a "thin" line or more of a "thick" grey area separating those who clearly are rational agents from those who are not. Being above or below it must correspond to some change in psychological capacities with plausible moral significance and which must be connected to an explanation of why the possession of certain capacities matters morally in the first place.

Traditional candidates for the specifically relevant capacity are rationality, self-consciousness, or autonomy. Whatever their merits, it is still true that they come in degrees and that some individuals possess them to a greater extent than others. So, if we hold a threshold view, we will reach what appears to be an arbitrary, i.e., unjustified, position.[15]

This can be observed by thinking of two individuals with almost exactly the same capacities. One of them has these capacities only to a slightly lower degree than the other, but the former falls below the threshold while the latter stands above. If arbitrariness is a good enough reason to reject a view, we should certainly reject this one. If, nevertheless, we remain

[14] The idea of range property has famously been introduced by John Rawls. See Rawls (1999 [1971], p. 444).

[15] It would be of no avail to claim that the threshold is vague and hence allows for an area of indeterminacy. As explained, the threshold is either a thin line (demarcating clear-cut cases) or a thick gray area (separating the sets of clear-cut cases by an area of indeterminacy). Given that psychological capacities are gradual, any thin line is unjustified. Nonetheless, if we accept a thick gray area, we are led to a regression to the first dilemma: Either there is a thin line that demarcates the clear-cut cases from the grey area or these are separated by a further area of indeterminacy. Thus, we are driven again to an infinite regress or to a thin line.

convinced that such capacities are relevant, regarding how equality and priority reasons apply to individuals, then we are led to accept the alternative view. We will thus have to conclude that because individuals differ in the degree to which they have these capacities, the strength of the equality and priority reasons that apply to each individual will have to be correspondingly adjusted. That is, one must reject that these principles apply equally to all individuals above certain cognitive capacities, such as those usually considered constitutive of rational agency.

At this point, supporters of the Exclusion Approach might accept this implication, thinking that the alternative – intervening in nature on behalf of wild animals – is too implausible.[16] Yet, on reflection, I believe that the consequences of endorsing that view might be unacceptable. This is particularly the case once we confront the question of whether the strength of equality and priority reasons also varies along the scale of net-negative well-being. Extending the variation of equality or priority reasons to net-negative well-being commits one to the claim that the moral importance of similar levels of net-negative well-being varies even among rational agents. For instance, it is more important to assist a certain rational agent and rescue them from a life not worth living than it is to assist another rational agent with a life similarly not worth living, simply because the second is endowed with lesser capacities.

Yet that still excludes less cognitively endowed individuals from the scope of distributive principles, even regarding the scale of net-negative well-being. Now, consider the following case:

> *The Saviors' Base:* Imagine a community where human beings leading wretched lives go to get assistance – the Saviors' Base. Some human beings that come to the Base possess complex cognitive capacities that set them above the threshold. Others are severely cognitively impaired human beings below the threshold. All those who do not receive assistance lead lives of net-negative well-being, though the lives of the cognitively impaired, when unassisted, are much worse than the lives of the better cognitively endowed.

According to the Exclusion Approach, the plight of the cognitively impaired humans, even if more terrible, should give way before the plight of the rational humans, which is given moral priority. This is highly problematic and would be found unacceptable even by many of those who might consider the Exclusion Approach intuitively plausible alongside

---

[16] This is the argumentative path Richard Arneson followed when I presented the aforementioned challenges to him on July 2014 at CEU Summer School. See also Arneson (2014).

the net-positive side of the scale.[17] But if that is so, then equality and priority reasons must apply, and to the same extent, to all sentient beings, irrespective of how sophisticated their cognitive capacities are, at least regarding levels of net-negative well-being.

What follows from this regarding animals living in the wild? Given the widespread presence of suffering in nature, wild animals are plausibly the worse-off individuals.

As we saw, it is extremely implausible that nonrational agents are also excluded from the scope of equality on the negative side of the scale of net well-being. Therefore, the net-negative levels of well-being experienced by nonhuman individuals are as morally important as similar levels that might be endured by severely cognitively impaired humans or by rational agents. The facts show how the level of net-negative well-being of nonhumans is high indeed, and their numbers are enormous (see Chapter 3). Thus, even after all these adjustments, the same implication follows – intervening on behalf of wild animals is a moral priority.

Finally, there is a further difficulty of threshold views worth discussing. The scale of rational agency capacities may continue to much higher degrees of psychological capacities than any human rational agent has ever, or perhaps will ever, possess. Indeed, the scale may go on indefinitely. It would not be surprising that, compared to other possible rational beings (even if not yet existing on Earth), human rational agents are rather on the lower sections of the scale.[18]

> *The posthumans*: Suppose that a group of human beings colonized planet X. Due to a process of progressive cognitive enhancement, they developed into beings with very high cognitive capacities. Compared to paradigmatic human beings on Earth, they might be considered posthumans. Now, suppose that these posthumans come to Earth to operate a massive transfer of resources from most human beings to most *posthumans*. What are we required to do?

On a threshold view, it would be suspicious that the line that separates those to whom equality and priority apply from those to whom it does not happens to coincide with the average cognitive capacities of human beings. It is possible that the line is much lower down the scale, just as it is possible that it is much higher up. That might, in fact, be the prevalent position

---

[17] Certainly, these implications would not be considered unacceptable under modal personism (Chapter 2) or relational approaches (Chapter 6). Nevertheless, as I have argued, I believe we should reject these views.

[18] For similar examples, see Nozick (1974, p. 41).

among posthumans. Thus, it is conceivable that human beings would also be excluded from the scope of equality and priority. If we assume that there is a threshold establishing a relevant moral demarcation between rational agents like us and other sentient beings, nothing bars in principle the possibility that there are more such thresholds up the scale of rational agency capacities. These posthumans might be one or several thresholds above us.

On these accounts, human rational agents stand to them as nonrational sentients stand to mere rational agents. Even if all led lives of net-negative well-being, the *posthumans* would not be required to perform sacrifices to assist them, for example, by preventing a massive shift of natural resources from most human beings to the *posthumans*. Given what it means for a human rational agent to lead a life of net-negative well-being, this implication seems unacceptable. As Richard Arneson himself acknowledges, "To put it mildly, these implications of the rational agency account are hard to swallow."[19]

It appears, then, that once one tries to fill in the details of the Exclusion Approach, one faces the prospect of denying equal consideration of interests even among those above the threshold. This seems hardly acceptable, especially when the levels of well-being of individuals are net negative. The contrary implies that the interests of cognitively impaired humans not to have miserable lives make very weak claims on us. Since that is highly implausible, one should conclude that all sentient beings should be considered within the scope of distributive principles, at least, again, on the net-negative scale. Since wild animals are very badly off, we have strong equality or priority reasons to act on their behalf. The Exclusion Approach does not successfully block intervention.

7.2   The Deflation Approach

Consider now the second strategy:

> *The Deflation Approach:* Equality- or priority-based reasons, when applied to sentient individuals with lower psychological capacities, are weaker than when applied to individuals with higher psychological capacities.

This strategy does not consist in excluding certain individuals from the scope of equality or priority. Rather, it purports to show how, even though distributive principles apply to all sentient individuals, they apply much

---

[19] Arneson (2014, p. 40).

less strongly to a certain subset of them. This is done by claiming that the currency of distribution is not individual well-being, but rather fortune, where "fortune" stands for well-being relativized to individual psycholog- ical capacities. This strategy is endorsed both by Jeff McMahan[20] and Peter Vallentyne,[21] albeit with certain differences.[22] It allows them to justify the claim that though nonhuman animals have extremely low levels of well- being, we are not required to carry out a massive transfer of resources so as to make them better off. In what follows, I will examine both versions of the Deflation Approach and assess the extent to which they might provide compelling reasons not to intervene for the sake of wild animals and for choosing other aims instead.

a) McMahan's Native Potential Account of Fortune

According to McMahan's Native Potential Account of Fortune, to be badly off means to be unfortunate, where misfortune is understood as a failure to realize one's native psychological capacities and potential.[23] On this account, an individual is more or less fortunate (they are better or worse off for the purposes of equality or priority) to the degree that their actual level of well-being is closer or further from their maximum level of well-being as determined by the highest capacities one ever has the native potential to achieve.[24] An individual's "genuinely native potential" is the one "grounded in [the individual's] physical constitution" "somehow present in the existing neural hardware." This should be distinguished from a broader notion of potential, which includes "all that a being could become, compatibly with preserving its identity by being externally augmented."[25]

Thus, to increase an individual's level of well-being does not necessarily imply that they are made better off (fortunate). In fact, so the argument goes, that will not be the case if their actual level of well-being is increased while their capacity and potential for well-being are enhanced. By modi- fying their maximum potential, such enhancement would change the

---

[20] McMahan (1996).   [21] Vallentyne (2005).

[22] For instance, Vallentyne believes that fortune so understood is the currency of both equality and priority. As mentioned, McMahan restricts it to the latter (1996, pp. 28–31), but for argumentative purposes it is possible to extend it as well to the former. I believe that nothing hinges on that.

[23] McMahan (1996, pp. 16–24).

[24] McMahan (1996:24). Thus, this account implies the following asymmetry: An accident that diminishes one's potential for well-being counts as a misfortune but to have one's capacities enhanced would not make one more fortunate.

[25] McMahan (1996: 22).

relevant scale for comparison of fortune. Because the scale has changed, the fact that an individual's well-being has increased does not imply that they are better off or more fortunate. That will only be so if their well-being is closer to their maximum native potential.

Thus, two important implications follow from McMahan's account:

(i)   We have no equality or priority reasons to enhance the potential for well-being of the congenitally less endowed individuals (human or nonhuman).

(ii) For any given level of well-being, an individual with a lower capacity or potential for well-being is better off than another individual with the same level but higher capacity or potential for well-being. For example, suppose that both Nico's and Kai's actual levels of well-being are 50. However, Nico's maximum capacity for well-being is 100, whereas Kai's is 150. On this view, Nico is more fortunate than Kai because they are closer to their maximum possible level of well-being.

Since implication (ii) is common to both McMahan and Vallentyne's accounts, I shall now focus on what is distinctive about McMahan's proposal and thus assess his rejection of our reasons to enhance the congenitally less endowed.

Consider the following scenarios in which there are certain treatments that can be given to two persons (call them Alex and Robin) affecting their capacities, their well-being, or both:

A.   Alex has average cognitive capacities but suffers an accident that renders them severely cognitively impaired. Because the impairment is accidental, their native maximum potential for well-being remains unchanged. However, *with or without treatment, their overall level of well-being will remain the same.*

According to McMahan's view, in both cases, that is, with or without treatment, they would be equally fortunate. Therefore, we do not have priority reasons to treat them.

B.   As in A, Alex has average cognitive capacities but suffers an accident that renders them severely cognitively impaired. Again, because the impairment is accidental, their native maximum potential for well-being remains unchanged, and there is a treatment that can restore their capacities. This time, *if treated, they will enjoy a greater level of well-being, one that would be closer to their maximum native potential.*

On McMahan's view, Alex will be better off or more fortunate if treated. This means that we have priority reasons to treat them.

C.   Robin suffers from a severe congenital cognitive impairment. However, there is a treatment that can enhance their capacities and potentials to the levels of an average human being. Whether they are treated or not, however, as in A, *their overall level of well-being will remain the same.*

Now, on McMahan's account, there are no priority reasons to treat Robin. This is not because in either way they will have the same level of well-being (as Alex in A). Rather, this is because we only have priority reasons to benefit someone when that will render their levels of well-being closer to their native maximum potential. In this case, treating Robin will not benefit them in that way. In fact, enhancement would make them more unfortunate. Notice, however, that those who don't accept the distinction between fortune and well-being would find McMahan's view at this point already slightly counterintuitive since "with or without treatment, their overall level of well-being will remain the same." They would say that they are equally fortunate, not more unfortunate.

D.   As in C, Robin suffers from a severe congenital cognitive impairment. There is a treatment that can enhance their capacities and potentials to the levels of an average human being. If treated, they will enjoy a greater level of well-being, though *the distance between their new level of well-being and their new maximum potential is the same as the distance that existed between their previous level of well-being and their maximum native potential.*

Again, on McMahan's view, there are no priority reasons to treat them, even though it is true that their well-being will increase. This is because, on this view, our reasons do not apply to enhance an individual's maximum potential for well-being, but only to raise their well-being within the scale of their maximum native potential.

E.   Robin suffers from a severe congenital cognitive impairment. Their potential is 10. Their current level of well-being now is 8. So, on McMahan's account, their total fortune is 8/10, which is 0.8. There is a treatment that can enhance their capacities and potentials to the levels of an average human being, say, 20. If they are treated, their overall level of well-being will be increased to 14. On the same account of fortune, *their resulting fortune after the treatment will be 14/20, which is 0.7.*

This example shows how under certain circumstances an increase in well-being can mean a decrease in fortune according to McMahan's account of it. Since 8 is higher relative to 10 (0.8) than 14 is relative to 20 (0.7), on McMahan's account we would have reasons *not* to treat them because that would be *worse* for them, as they would be less fortunate. That seems very implausible since their well-being will be far greater.

Now, while the Native Potential Account of Fortune provides an acceptable solution for A–C that is not the case with D and E. As in B, in both D and E, the treatment is worthwhile because it increases somebody's well-being. In addition, the patients' interest in improving their well-being is the same in B, D, and E, and our reasons to treat them are as strong as our reasons to do it in B. Yet the Native Potential Account implies that the latter is false.

Nevertheless, if what matters is how our choices affect the interests of individuals and that does not vary across the scenarios we are considering here, our reasons cannot vary merely because the patients' psychological capacities do. This must be the case independently of how their well-being is improved, be it through cognitive enhancement or otherwise. This shows that the proposal falls prey of highly counterintuitive results.[26]

This suggests that, at the very least, McMahan's account of fortune should be revised so as to relativize the well-being of an individual, at some time, to the psychological capacities and potential of that individual at that time, whether that potential is congenital or not.[27] But these examples perhaps show as well that the relativization requirement should be entirely abandoned.[28] This point may be strengthened if we consider a veil of

---

[26] To be sure McMahan allows that there may be further reasons of beneficence to protect and care for the "cognitively impaired" and nonhuman animals. He claims, "They are not, of course, our only moral reasons to protect and care for the cognitively impaired. Simple beneficence requires that we take due account of the interests of the cognitively impaired, just as it requires that we respect the similar interests of animals. In the case of the cognitively impaired, however, these reasons are supplemented by further reasons to respect the commitments of those persons who are specially related to them" (1996:34–35).

[27] That would render McMahan's proposal almost identical to Vallentyne's.

[28] In addition, it might be argued that if we accept that nonhumans have a lower potential for positive well-being than humans, then they plausibly have a lower potential for negative well-being. This means that if a nonhuman and a human animal have net-negative levels of well-being, that is worse in the case of a nonhuman animal. That is, someone with a net-negative level of -2 and a negative potential of -4 is, by symmetry, more unfortunate than someone with a net-negative level of -2 and a negative potential of -40. Suppose this is not so and negative levels of well-being are just considered with regard to positive potential. We get the same result: The nonhuman animal has an actual well-being of -2 and a potential of 4, their fortune is $-2/4$. The human has a well-being of -2 and a potential of 40, their fortune is $-2/40$. $-2/4$ is a much more negative result than $-2/40$. Thus, on McMahan's account, negative well-being is much worse if your potential is smaller. Accepting McMahan's account means we should regard what happens in the wild, where huge

ignorance argument in which we could decide the potential for well-being of each individual that will exist in the world without knowing our place in it. It seems that we would surely favor a world where everyone enjoyed equal capacity and potential for well-being. At least, insofar we think that impartiality must be one of the features of principles of distributive justice.

b) Vallentyne's Fortune Relative to Moral Standing

Peter Vallentyne[29] acknowledges that equality and priority apply to all sentient animals. This is not equivalent, however, to the claim that equality- and priority-based reasons apply to all of them with the same strength. If they did, he acknowledges, a massive shift of resources (or well-being) would be required from most humans to most nonhuman animals since the latter are worse off. Yet, Vallentyne claims, it would be unreasonable to endorse such implication, which he dubs "the Problematic Conclusion." The strength of equality and priority reasons when applied to nonhuman animals must be somehow deflated.

Vallentyne deviates from McMahan's account given the possibility of what he calls *radical enhancement*, that is, the technological upgrade of individuals' potential for well-being irrespective of their species. Under this assumption, it is conceivable to reach a point where everyone's potential for well-being is the same across species. Thus, for the purposes of distributive principles, the moral standing of an individual must be determined by their capacity for well-being (currently realized ability), rather than by their potential (currently unrealized ability).

He says,

> I shall suggest that fortune should be understood as wellbeing relativized to the degree of moral standing, where moral standing is grounded in the capacities of the individuals (rather than in their potentials).[30]

Since, unlike McMahan's, Vallentyne's account does not require the relevant capacities to be congenital, it leaves open the possibility that equality or priority may demand us the enhancement of the less congenitally psychologically endowed, when that will make them better off.[31]

---

numbers of animals have net-negative lives, as a much more serious issue than if humans were in the same situation.

[29] Vallentyne (2005).   [30] Ibid, p.28.

[31] Indeed, according to Vallentyne, there are certain circumstances in which enhancement might be required, for instance, when for contingent reasons it's not possible to equalize fortune among different individuals in a scenario without enhancing some of them (2005:431–432).

While rejecting (i) the claim that we lack equality and priority reasons to enhance the less congenitally psychologically endowed, this account still implies (ii). That is, a low level of net-positive well-being for an individual with a low capacity for well-being is less important for the purposes of equality and priority than a similar level of a better endowed individual. This is so because, on Vallentyne's calculus, the former might be as equally or even more fortunate than the latter.[32]

What equality and priority require of us is, thus, less stringent the lower an individual's capacity for well-being is. Even if nonhuman animals have lower levels of well-being, they are not necessarily worse off since their psychological capacities are so much lower than those of average humans. Accordingly, what we owe to nonhuman animals for the purposes of distribution is significantly reduced.

Applied to the case of wild animals, Vallentyne's argument might thus be synthesized as follows:

(i)   The currency of distribution is fortune, where fortune is well-being relativized to moral standing.

(ii)   A lower capacity for well-being implies lower moral standing.

(iii) Most nonhuman animals have a lower capacity for well-being. Hence, they have lower moral standing.

(iv)   Therefore, most nonhuman animals are not worse off than most humans.

(v)   If (iv), then we have no equality and priority reasons (or only very weak ones) to significantly shift benefits from most humans to most nonhuman animals, including to those living in the wild.

(vi)   Thus, intervention on behalf of wild animals is almost never required.

An immediate way to answer this is to accept Vallentyne's argument while only dedicating a certain amount of resources to help wild animals. In this way, the view would not oppose helping wild animals, not even significantly doing so, but merely undertaking a massive transfer of resources from most humans to most nonhuman animals. There are, however,

---

[32] This makes Vallentyne's view sound like Raz's view of the diminishing significance of well-being (Raz 1986, Chapter 9). There, Raz treats the reason-giving force of the provision of a unit of well-being to depend on the level of advantage of the recipient. But instead of focusing on how close the recipient is to the zero level, he focuses on how far they are to the satiation point where their life cannot be improved. On this view, when individuals have different satiation points, the individuals with the higher satiation points have stronger claims because the distance between their actual level and their satiated level is bigger.

other, stronger grounds on which to reject Vallentyne's attempt to escape the so-called "Problematic Conclusion."[33]

First, if the strength of equality and priority reasons is gradual and is to be adjusted following variations in psychological capacities, it must be gradual *throughout*. The psychological capacities on which the capacity for well-being supervenes vary among human beings. If that is so, the strength of our equality and priority reasons must vary as well. If we conceive of how well or badly off an individual is as their level of well-being relativized to their capacities, then for each individual we will have to assess their capacities and derive our reasons accordingly.

The Deflation Approach implies that the strength of equality- and priority-based reasons vary even among rational agents, depending on the sophistication of their capacity for well-being. In addition, the problem cannot be solved by retreating to a threshold view since all such boundaries ultimately prove arbitrary.

Moreover, even if it were accepted that these considerations apply to the net-positive side of the scale of well-being, it is highly implausible that they apply to the net-negative side as well. Consider again *the Saviors' Base*. Vallentyne's proposal would also imply that the net-negative well-being of cognitively impaired human beings counts for much less than similar levels of negative well-being of non-impaired humans. Hence, we should prioritize assistance to the latter. It would also imply that the moral importance of net-negative levels of well-being of the least endowed rational agents counts for less than other best endowed rational agents with similar levels of well-being. Nevertheless, that would justify unacceptable practices such as the sacrifice of the least endowed for the benefit of the most endowed individuals.[34]

Finally, a problem similar to the *posthumans* also follows for the Deflation Account. We may imagine sentient beings with a high capacity for well-being, such that average human beings stand to them as most nonhuman animals stand to average human beings. Equality and priority reasons would then apply to these superior beings much more strongly than to average humans. Even if humans were in such appalling conditions as most nonhumans currently are, no massive shift of resources for their

---

[33] For further criticisms, see Holtug (2007).
[34] On moderate versions of prioritarianism, it might sometimes be justified to sacrifice the interests of the worse off provided that the benefit to the better off is substantial enough. However, in the cases we are dealing with here, the benefits in terms of well-being for the most endowed would be as large as the benefits from which the least endowed are deprived.

benefit would be morally required from these superior beings. This would certainly be unacceptable.

However, if we reject this, it is dubious that we can avoid that a massive shift of resources is morally required for the benefit of nonhuman animals. This is so because plausibly animals are currently the worse-off individuals due to their high levels of net-negative well-being, particularly, those living in the wild (see Chapter 3). As the scenarios considered above show, this is a conclusion we would fully embrace if the worse-off individuals belonged to the human species. Again, we should be wary of speciesist bias in assessing our conclusions. Once we get rid of it, the so-called "problematic conclusion" may just be the "equitable conclusion" after all. And if that is so, then the Deflation Approach (McMahan or Vallentyne's version) cannot successfully show that intervention on behalf of animals is not a moral priority. Moreover, it is important to stress that even if we accept this approach and the interests of wild animals count for very little in comparison to humans, given their huge numbers, they will still count enough for us to ought to help them.

7.3 The Perfectionist Approach

A third approach to the problem at hand is quite different from the previous two.

> *The Perfectionist Approach*: A change that brings a great net increase in subjective welfare to those who are affected by it is a change for the worse if it involves the loss of one of "the best things in life."[35]

The best things in life are, according to Parfit, "the best kinds of creative activity and aesthetic experience, the best relationships between different people, and the other things which do most to make life worth living." Suppose that we are in a position in which we can significantly benefit a great number of individuals but can only do so through a massive transfer of resources that will expectably make it impossible to generate many of the "best things in life." This is the kind of choice we may be facing when considering intervening in nature.

So, applied to our case, the perfectionist argument could be formulated as follows:

(i) Intervention on behalf of animals comes at the cost of reducing or losing "the best things in life."

---

[35] See Parfit (2004 [1986], p. 19).

(ii)   Intervention on behalf of animals would significantly increase their
        levels of subjective welfare.
(iii)   Reduction or losses of "the best things in life" cannot be compen-
        sated by any benefits in terms of nonhuman subjective welfare.
(iv)   Therefore, intervention is not a moral priority. We must prioritize
        the pursuit and preservation of "the best things in life" rather than
        significantly benefit nonhuman animals.

Perfectionism is open to many challenges, though a general assessment of
its faults lies outside the scope of this book. Rather, I will focus on two
main worries that arise for a specific form of perfectionism – the one
endorsed by Parfit *and* here reconstructed as an attempt to ground a
priority objection to intervention. Parfit's view is characterized in terms
of the achievement or realization of "the best things in life." These should
be understood as those kinds of things that, besides contributing the most
to make life worth living (having very high personal value), also have very
high impersonal value.

a)   Inegalitarian Implications for Distributive Purposes

According to the Perfectionist Approach, an outcome A is worse than an
outcome B if A involves the loss of objective goods, independently of how
A and B may stand with regard to subjective welfare. Now suppose that
A involves the loss of Venice[36] but as a result Alex and Robin are equally
better off. B does not involve such a loss. Alex is as well off as they would
have been in A though Robin is much worse off than Alex. Yet according
to the perfectionist, we should prioritize outcome B over A. That is, even
though no one is better off in B, and there is inequality resulting from
someone being worse off, B is considered better overall because there is no
loss of objective goods – Venice still exists.

Now consider a slightly different scenario:

> *The perfection monster.*[37] Imagine a scenario in which a cognitively well-
> endowed being is able to bring about outstanding creative activity and
> aesthetic experience, inaccessible to average human beings. So that the
> monster remains productive, it must receive enormous amounts of

---

[36] An example of objective good, according to Parfit, ibid.

[37] Someone might say that great suffering is a price that is worth paying for a world with alleged
objective goods present in nature, such as the beauty and elegance of predation. On this
understanding, perfectionism might be better considered under the Jeopardy heading. But as
argued in Chapter 5, objections to intervention from jeopardy also fail.

resources. Shifting such resources toward them means many humans having merely worth living lives, rather than lives at much higher levels of subjective welfare.

According to the Perfectionist approach, we are committed to accepting a scenario in which the Perfection monster receives all the resources and gets to realize these objective goods even though everyone else will be affected for the worse. We are also committed to agreeing that a scenario in which all human beings are much better off but the Perfection Monster lacks resources for creative activity is worse than a scenario in which they do so at the expense of everyone else being worse off.

What the Venice example and the Perfection Monster experiment reveal is the highly inegalitarian implications of the Perfectionist Approach, which renders it unacceptable to most of us.

Yet the counterintuitive results of the approach become even more apparent when considering scenarios that involve not only inequality but net-negative levels of subjective welfare.[38] Roger Crisp, for example, who is not an egalitarian, would not sacrifice a pristine rainforest for the sake of equality above a sufficiency threshold, but he would sacrifice it to prevent suffering or the risk of humanity falling below sufficiency.[39] If we reject speciesism, it seems the same should apply in the case of nonhuman animals. This unwelcome implication is, in fact, something of which Parfit was well aware.

b) The Moral Importance of Relieving or Preventing Great Suffering

Parfit claims,

> We should reject the Nietzschean view that the prevention of great suffering can be ranked wholly below the preservation of creation of the best things in life. What should Perfectionists claim about great suffering? But this problem is irrelevant here, since we can assume that in the various outcomes we are considering there would be no such suffering.[40]

Two crucial implications follow from this. First, the Perfectionist Approach is an account that works, at best (and not without committing us to

---

[38] Thomas Nagel, for instance, declares not to favor equality if it comes at the expense of haute cuisine, fine art, and a number of goods that possess what he calls "excellence" to a degree that makes us morally required to preserve them (1991). It seems reasonable to assume that the majority of us would clearly reject that this justifies letting other individuals to live lives barely worth living or, as in the case of huge numbers of animals suffering in nature, not worth living at all.

[39] See Crisp (1994).   [40] Parfit (2004 [1986], p. 20).

unwelcome inegalitarian scenarios),[41] when exclusively considering out-comes with only net-positive levels of subjective welfare. Second, even if we bite the bullet and accept the inegalitarian implications of the Perfectionist Approach, we are nevertheless committed, on Parfit's view, to accepting that the pursuit of objective goods does not have moral priority over the prevention or alleviation of great suffering.

But if the relief of great suffering should have precedence over the preservation of any such objective goods, then the Perfectionist Argument against intervention collapses. The vast majority of wild animals likely have lives of net suffering. Failing to intervene on behalf of animals on a perfectionist basis amounts to prioritizing the pursuit and preservation of "the best things in life" over the prevention or alleviation of great suffering.

Plausibly enough, on Parfit's view, the realization of objective goods cannot have moral priority over the prevention of great suffering. But in that case, failure to intervene on behalf of wild animals cannot be justified on perfectionist grounds.[42]

In addition, even if we accept the priority of promoting "the best things in life" that would still not amount to opposing helping wild animals. It would merely restrict a prohibition to help, conditional to reducing the best things in life. Yet, it would be perfectly acceptable to help animals at the expense of reducing only secondary things in life. Moreover, helping others in need may plausibly qualify as one of "the best things in life." Many character-based ethicists would agree that in addition to sophisti-cated pleasures one might selfishly pursue, there must be other, more meaningful elements among "the best things in life." Perhaps Gandhi was enjoying some of the best things in life while pursuing justice in extremely impoverished conditions – a "good" that millionaires are unable to access. If this is plausible, then, by engaging in altruistic behavior like helping wild animals, we may be promoting the presence of "excellent goods" that make our lives much better and richer.

---

[41] Some would say that it is the price to pay to block the Repugnant Conclusion. See Parfit (1984, 2004 [1986]).

[42] Someone might object to this that even though nonintervention cannot always be justified on perfectionist grounds, there are nevertheless at least one kind of cases in which it would be so. This is when intervention would improve the lives of animals but these would still have lives not worth living. Nevertheless, that would not be so. Even if the benefit of intervention for present animals would be negligible, the implication is that we should devote resources to research better ways in which to intervene in the future. If we do so, there are many individuals in the future with lives of net suffering that will not exist and many individuals who will instead have lives of net-positive subjective welfare.

Until now, I examined different arguments against intervention in nature based on priority considerations. They all have the same conclusion, which is that intervening to benefit wild animals should not be favored over other courses of action that bring about more moral value. The reasons why they reach this conclusion diverge. On the Exclusion Approach, this is because wild animals fall outside the scope of distributive principles, whereas most human beings are within such scope. On the Deflation Approach, this is because, since wild animals have a lower capacity for well-being (and thus have lower moral standing), increasing their well-being produces less moral value. Finally, on the Perfectionist Approach, this is because increasing the well-being (taken as subjective welfare) of nonhuman animals cannot compensate for the loss of objective goods involved in doing so. I concluded that none of these approaches could successfully present a case against intervention. They all have unacceptable results. This is particularly true regarding those scenarios that involve net-negative levels of subjective welfare. In such cases, it is very hard to believe that our moral priority is not to prevent or relieve great suffering, even if those affected are nonhuman individuals.

Notice that this analysis is intended as an assessment of potential objections based on the scope of certain principles of justice, though remaining neutral with regard to the existence of obligations of justice toward wild animals. My point may be formulated as a conditional: *If* one claims that improving human well-being has priority over intervening in nature for the sake of nonhuman animals because equality and priority reasons either (a) do not apply to wild animals or (b) are significantly weaker, *then* we will necessarily run into morally unacceptable scenarios, thereby failing to successfully object to intervention in nature.

7.4 Domesticated Animals First

Now, another way of conceiving the Priority Objection would be to claim something along the following lines:

> *Domesticated animals first:* When confronted with the choice between intervening in nature on behalf of wild animals and benefiting domesticated animals (particularly, farmed animals), the latter has priority over the former.

The spirit of the objection is embraced by different pro-animal scholars and activists, though the reasons for endorsing it may differ. The arguments supporting the objection usually fall under two broad categories: (a)

arguments based on the alleged greater strictness of negative duties and (b)
arguments based on the effectiveness of strategies to ameliorate the plight
of nonhuman animals. Regarding (a), the view has recently been articu-
lated by Kyle Johannsen,[43] according to whom "[h]arms to domesticated
animals involve a violation of negative duties, while allowing harm [to wild
animals] does not." Since "[n]egative duties are typically weightier than
positive duties," fulfilling our negative duties to alleviate harms to domesticated animals has priority over fulfilling our positive duties to alleviate
harms to wild animals.[44]

Many are inclined to agree that if an agent plays a causal role in bringing
about a harmful state of affairs, then they have a greater responsibility to
prevent or otherwise mitigate its effects than if they were an innocent
bystander. Yet, that does not entail that not harming has priority over
helping. Or, in other words, negative duties are weightier than positive
duties. It simply entails that, sometimes, negative duties may provide us
with additional reasons to alleviate harms. This is crucial since having an
additional reason not to harm does not necessarily lead to having stronger
reasons not to harm across the board. That reason will have to be weighed
against the reasons we have to help, and its additional force may turn out
to be negligible. At any rate, the balance of reasons cannot be settled by
simply assuming that reasons for helping are weaker than reasons for not
harming. That would be, as some have pointed out, question begging.[45]

In addition, our intuitions in relevant cases also fail to support (a).
Consider the following reconstruction of a trolley problem: Imagine that
pushing a lever causes a railway train to steer down track A upon which a
nonhuman animal is tied, while not pushing it allows you to remain on
track B upon which another nonhuman animal is tied. If (a) were correct,
then your reasons to proceed down on track B would be stronger than your
reasons to steer down A. Remaining on track B allows you to better fulfill
your duty not to cause harm while steering down track A does not.
However, it seems reasonable to predict that most people's intuitions
would tell them that it would make no difference which alternative you
adopt. If this is right, then the evaluative judgment of the alternatives
should be symmetrical. This suggests that the distinction between causing
harm and allowing harm bears much less significance than is usually
assumed and that the claim that avoiding harms to exploited animals has
priority over helping wild animals cannot be grounded on (a).

[43] Johannsen (2020).   [44] Ibid, p. 87.   [45] Lichtenberg (2010).

Finally, even though my goal is not to make a political case for helping wild animals, I would like to briefly tackle Johannsen's claim that "state provided assistance to wild animals must be democratically enacted if it's to be legitimate." This is because "fulfilling our collective negative duties to domesticated animals is arguably a requirement of legitimacy," while "fulfilling our collective positive duties to wild animals is not."[46] I believe that Johannsen's position again begs the question about the higher strictness of negative duties as well as relies on a narrow conception of political legitimacy, one that squares political coercion with the harm principle. Once we realize that the moral distinction between negative duties and positive duties is much less sharp than originally thought, the priority of a harm principle (prohibition to wrongly making someone worse off) over a benefit principle (prohibition to wrongly failing to make someone better off) loses its force.

Alternatively, one might adopt a Samaritan model of political legitimacy, according to which the state is permitted to do whatever is necessary to save others from facing the perilous circumstances of the state of nature without imposing an unreasonable cost.[47] A model of political legitimacy which is sensitive to the moral significance of samaritanism in this way entails that the state has a right to force in the absence of consent and despite dissent. Coercion is permitted because the peril of others generates weightier moral reasons. And even if it may be true that samaritanism does not imply "anything like a full-blown liberal welfare state,"[48] it is plausible to think that it can be expanded to justify ensuring that most vulnerable individuals have their basic needs met.[49] Crucially, a Samaritan duty binds us to help others in need *anywhere*.[50] Thus, fulfilling our duties to help wild animals might be as much a requirement of legitimacy as fulfilling our negative duties to domesticated animals.

Now, regarding (b), Yew-Kwang Ng[51] articulates the intuition that we should focus on farmed animals as a matter of near-term strategy. The reasons invoked are (i) causal responsibility for harm making someone more likely to be persuaded to minimize it; (ii) our limited knowledge on how to help wild animals today; and (iii) the potential risk of currently focusing on wild animal suffering. Since interventions to help wild animals could have long-term ecological repercussions, we should defer measures to help them until a better informed future. In Ng's words, "after much

---

[46] Johannsen (2020, p. 92).   [47] Wellman (1996, 2001).   [48] Wellman (2001, 757–758).
[49] Delmas (2014a).   [50] Delmas (2014b).   [51] Ng (2016).

greater concern for farmed animals has become the norm, legally and culturally."[52]

As I have argued elsewhere[53] regarding (i), it is not clear that causal responsibility for harm makes someone more likely to be persuaded to minimize it, or to stop it altogether, as Ng suggests. In the case of harms to domesticated animals, given deep-seated psychological biases,[54] people may be less prone to undertake big changes in their daily habits, such as the food they eat. On the other hand, concern for wild animals does not have such a salient impact on our daily practices. Hence people might be more inclined to act on it. As for (ii), besides ways of helping wild animals already available on a micro or medium scale (e.g., as rescues, medical intervention to help the injured, vaccination programs), ignorance regarding large-scale interventions to reduce wild animal suffering is not a rationale for emphasizing the suffering of farmed animals over the suffering of those living in the wild. If, as Ng claims, due to their high numbers, wild animals are much more important in the long term, what seems to follow is to promote the requisite research for potential future evidence-based interventions to help them. (This point is developed at length in Chapter 8.)

Finally, (iii) the mere fact that a certain intervention in nature presents a risk in terms of long-term ecological repercussions is, in itself, neither positive nor negative. That would depend on whether its effects on wild animals are, overall, beneficial or detrimental to their well-being. At any rate, even if one conceded that intervening now would, on many occasions, harm wild animals more than it would help them, it would still not follow that our focus should be predominantly on farmed animals. Again, given the long-term importance of wild animal suffering, that would give us very strong reasons to do research on how to make it more feasible to carry out future long-term sustained interventions to benefit wild animals. In addition, if it were true that concern for farmed animals led to concern for wild animal suffering, one might confidently expect to find great concern for wild animal suffering among, for instance, animal ethicists. Nevertheless, with very few exceptions, animal ethicists usually fail to see those wild animals in need as an object of moral concern. And even if Ng is right that raising awareness of farmed animal suffering will increase long-term concern for wild animal suffering, it does not follow that people will recognize that there is also reason to intervene in nature to help. Awareness also needs to be raised about how animals fare in the wild, by showing the

---

[52] Ng (2016, p. 7).   [53] Faria (2016).   [54] See, for example, Rothgerber (2020).

evidence that counters the idyllic view of nature. People will care about wild animals only to the extent that they know the truth about their suffering. For instance, in a study carried out by Animal Charity Evaluators, people exposed to an environmental rationale for reducing the consumption of animal products were shown to be less supportive of intervening in nature to alleviate wild animal suffering, plausibly influenced by the belief that wild animals typically lead good lives in nature.[55] It is thus crucial that we be careful in designing our strategy, in a way that is both sensitive to human attitudes, biases, and beliefs about animals in nature and transformative to our current understanding of human-wild animal relations.[56]

Moreover, I believe that the tension between alleviating harms to domesticated animals and alleviating harms to wild animals is more theoretical than practical. This is because refraining from doing harmful things does not usually conflict with doing beneficial things we have not been doing and vice-versa. Helping a drowning child in a pond does not normally constitute an obstacle to refraining from beating them. Likewise, helping wild animals suffering from, say, an infectious disease is not in tension with stopping from participating in the suffering caused by industrial animal agriculture. Moreover, many actions may in fact help achieve both aims. Spreading the idea that we should reduce wild animal disease is likely to benefit domesticated animals as well, insofar as the reasons for doing it are anchored in the moral relevance of nonhuman welfare and *not* on the agent's causal role in diminishing it. The opposite however is not likely to occur. At any rate, whenever these aims clash (if at all), I think the latter should take priority, given considerations of scale and, especially, neglectedness. This last point will be explored in Chapter 8.

[55] Animal Charity Evaluators (2016a).   [56] Waldhorn 2019.

CHAPTER 8

Tractability

Let us assume now that many people are persuaded by the moral priority of reducing wild animal suffering. Still, some might say that it is not an issue worth acting on because we have no idea how to put it into practice. In other words, wild animal suffering is intractable. Tractability is one of the key components of the three-factor framework used to rank focus areas.[1] The framework may be fleshed out as follows:

(i)   Importance: What is the scale of the problem in the area?
(ii) Tractability: How solvable is the problem in the area?
(iii) Neglectedness: How neglected is the area?

Many working on cause-prioritization are convinced that wild animal suffering scores high at both (i) and (iii). This is because it is an issue that could positively affect an extraordinary number of individuals with very few resources being allocated to it. With regard to (ii), however, they are unsure. That is, it remains unclear whether there are "definite interventions for progress within this cause, with strong evidence behind them."[2]

> *Tractability Objection*: We have decisive reasons not to intervene in nature because wild animal suffering is intractable.[3]

As supporters of the view argue, this is because of the epistemic difficulties associated with large-scale interventions to prevent wild animal suffering: "The nature of ecosystems leaves us with no reason to predict that interventions would reduce, rather than exacerbate, suffering" such that "there is at present, and for the foreseeable future, no reason to believe that the practical constraint on interventions is satisfied."[4]

By relying on human epistemic limitations and their associated risks, this challenge to intervention clearly echoes with the Perversity Objection

---

[1] MacAskill (2015).   [2] Todd (2013).   [3] Delon and Purves (2018).   [4] Ibid, p. 244.

already addressed in Chapter 4. But, as said, human beings are not in principle incapable of obtaining the necessary knowledge about possible net-positive interventions in the wild. This is even more so given the possibilities of future scientific and technological developments. If current knowledge is insufficient, then the clear answer seems to be that we ought to put more research into it (I will return to this point below).

8.1 Tractability and Feasibility

Tractability is often put together with feasibility though they should be distinguished. A problem is intractable if and only if there is no efficient (or reasonable time) solution to it. Often, problems thought to be intractable are not. World poverty or climate change are usually thought to fall under this category. But even conceding that it might be true of some hard cases, it would still not mean that all instances of the problem are equally hard to tackle. We can, for instance, select special cases or small problem sizes and work on finding approximate, near-optimal solutions. Even computationally intractable problems are often solved through heuristics or approximations so as to overcome the search costs associated with exhaustive approaches.[5] Indeed, many intractable problems are approximable, meaning there is an efficient method that produces an approximate result guaranteed to be within a certain range of values around the optimal solution.[6] A problem may be tractable though, and its current optimal solution infeasible. Something is infeasible if, and only if, it is practically impossible to achieve given certain facts about the world.[7]

This is, in fact, what the proponents of the Tractability Objection seem to have in mind by proposing a way forward. They say, "to justify interventions to prevent WAS [wild animal suffering], we need to develop models that predict the effects of interventions on biodiversity, ecosystem functioning, and animals' well-being."[8] But then, and contrary to their claim, wild animal suffering is *not* intractable. At most, and currently, large-scale interventions to prevent wild animal suffering are infeasible.

This shows that the alleged intractability thesis is, after all, a thesis about the low tractability of wild animal suffering equated with the infeasibility of large-scale interventions. But of course, the infeasibility of large-scale

---

[5] Cirillo and Valencia (2018). [6] I thank Carlos Castillo for bringing this to my attention.

[7] These facts are commonly thought to be logical consistency, nonviolation of the laws of nature, fixed history of the world, and human ability (Jensen 2009), though different views may privilege some facts over others.

[8] Delon and Purves (2018, p. 257).

interventions, if at all, does not imply that wild animal suffering is impossible to address. Carefully chosen small-scale interventions such as rescuing, vaccinating, or helping animals in natural disasters are likely to significantly improve the lives of animals without significant risk of negative side effects.

Against this it might be objected that our capacity to effectively have an impact on wild animal well-being is currently so limited that such low-impact interventions would be futile. Yet the rescue of animal victims of natural catastrophes such as the recent fires in Australia or the vaccination of animals against rabies, tuberculosis, and other diseases in Europe and North America[9] and of chimpanzees against polio in Congo[10] can hardly be claimed to have had no impact on the affected animals' well-being. Preventing them from experiencing the suffering caused by natural catastrophes or illnesses can only be beneficial to them. In fact, alleviating some of those forms of suffering may have increased their levels of well-being such that some of them crossed the threshold from having lives not worth living to lives minimally worth living.

These reasons for beneficial intervention exist even if it is true that for most animals the best state of affairs would have been one in which they had not come into existence. Supposing that only two scenarios were available for us – one in which (a) there was a small improvement in wild animal well-being and (b) the current state of affairs – we would still have reasons to prefer (a) over (b). With regard to wild animal suffering, it is crucial to assess the expected value of an intervention, such as in any other issue, in terms of harm reduction and not in terms of harm eradication.

Thus, after examination, the Tractability Objection – more accurately understood as a claim about feasibility – cannot provide sufficiently strong reasons for preferring the status quo over an alternative state of affairs. Hence, it should be rejected.

8.2 Neglectedness

Moreover, we know that the tractability of a problem, as understood within the above-mentioned importance–tractability–neglectedness framework, is significantly affected by neglectedness. Wild animal suffering is a typical uncrowded cause. Even though the tide is recently changing, there are very few academics as well as advocates working on this topic. Two honorable exceptions of organizations tackling the problem of wild animal

---

[9] MacInnes and LeBer (2000); Slate et al. (2005); Garrido et al. (2011).   [10] Goodall (1986, p. 58).

suffering are Animal Ethics and Wild Animal Initiative. If we added more resources into it, we could reasonably expect more opportunities for progress. That is, regarding those kinds of intervention that are currently infeasible, we have reasons to invest resources in developing new ways that enable us to assist wild animals in the future. Thus, a crucial way to increase the tractability of wild animal suffering is indirectly by working on its neglectedness. This could be done in a number of different ways.

Welfare Biology

As said, many important problems that humanity faces appear to be intractable. Yet they are not. Rather, they have not been previously formulated and researched scientifically. The development of welfare biology could give us precisely that with regard to wild animal suffering. Welfare biology is a proposed field of research that can be defined as the study of sentient organisms with respect to their well-being.[11] One might think that this work is already being done by conservation biology, but that would be misguided. The aim of conservation biology is the preservation of the Earth's biodiversity, its species and ecosystems, and nature as a whole. Preserving such entities is not only distinct from promoting individuals' well-being but often incompatible with it.[12]

Welfare biology is also distinct from compassionate conservation. Compassionate conservation has recently been proposed as an alternative to conventional conservation with a view to overcoming its disregard of the harms inflicted on individual wild animals, hence, heralding a more peaceful coexistence between humans and nonhumans.[13] Though a significant improvement, compassionate conservation is a model of inquiry still limited by an exclusive concern for anthropogenic harms. Welfare biology overcomes this important shortcoming by aiming to study all events that may negatively affect wild animal welfare, in particular, naturogenic phenomena.

As the study of the circumstances that affect nonhuman well-being in the wild, welfare biology could develop from an intersection between animal welfare science – expanding it to cover harms to animals not induced by human agency – and ecology, by focusing on the study of

---

[11] Ng (1995), Faria and Horta (2020), Soryl et al. (2020).
[12] Shelton (2004), Horta (2010d), Faria and Paez (2019).
[13] See, for example, Bekoff (2010, 2013); Ramp and Bekoff (2015); Gray (2017, 2018); For criticism, see, for instance, Griffin et al. (2020) and Coghlan and Cardilini (2021).

animal well-being within ecosystems. A compelling starting point would be to work on which currently undertaken interventions in nature are unintentionally beneficial for nonhuman animals. Salient examples include medium-scale vaccination programs, management of urban or peri-urban animal populations through contraception, health care interventions, food provision, or the protection of large herbivores, such as elephants.

Let us focus on the latter example. Elephants, unlike most wild animals, have large lifespans, very few offspring, high parental investment, and, as a consequence, high survival rates. They also consume a huge quantity of biomass,[14] thus preventing both smaller animals with larger progenies from coming into existence and large trophic chains from emerging within an ecosystem. This means that ecosystems where elephants are present are likely to contain lower levels of suffering.

Welfare biology has the potential to inform and expand policies of this kind that can have a beneficial effect not only on the targeted animals (e.g., elephants) but also on other animals indirectly affected by such policies. Consequently, research in welfare biology could make wild animal suffering an increasingly tractable cause area both by developing increasingly feasible ways to help wild animals and by indirectly raising interest in, and awareness of, wild animal suffering.

The previous point should not be seen as controversial since the most influential accounts of feasibility are conditional. That is, feasibility is to be understood as a function of the likelihood of success of an agent bringing about a certain state of affairs *conditional on trying*.[15] Clearly, the fact that people or collective agents may not be sufficiently motivated to carry out actions to relieve world poverty or mitigate the negative impact of climate change does not mean that it is infeasible for them to do so. Likewise, the fact that experts and people in general may be unlikely to research into reducing wild animal suffering does not mean that it is infeasible for them to bring about that state of affairs, *should they try*. Otherwise, if taken unconditionally, feasibility would simply be tantamount to reinforcing the status quo. As Anca Gheaus points out,

> I assume that, at all times, there are cases (...) that we individually or collectively cannot do anything about. One reason for this is the limitation of human knowledge at that moment. But, of course, we can invest our time, money, energy and thought in finding ways to change what is feasible. I also assume (...) that it is impossible to say in advance what will and what

---

[14] Guldemond and Aarde (2008). See also Pearce (2015).
[15] Gilabert and Lawford-Smith (2012). For an overview, see Erman and Möller (2020).

will not become feasible in the future, if enough resources are directed towards achieving a particular goal. In other words, we should be very careful with declaring something impossible in principle as opposed to infeasible in the light of current knowledge.[16]

This stresses yet another important point about feasibility: its diachronic nature. That is to say, the set of interventions and outcomes that qualify as feasible significantly changes over time. This is particularly true when considering collective action such that "many of the actions and outcomes that are not feasible for certain agents at particular times are nevertheless feasible for collective agents over time."[17]

Some might challenge this by saying that even if it is the case that cultural, institutional, economic, psychological, and motivational constraints are likely to be overcome by future collective action, it will be nevertheless impossible to lift persistent hard constraints.[18] Such is the case, so the argument might go, of interventions that defy the laws of nature such as potential large-scale interventions to reduce wild animal suffering, say for instance, through gene editing of r-strategists[19] or of large carnivores.[20]

There is significant disagreement as to whether laws of ecology, for instance, qualify as laws of nature at all, as say, compared to laws of physics.[21] But regardless of this, the argument seems to assume an erroneous view about the fixed structure of nature in general upon which human beings would be, by definition, incapable of interfering with. As discussed at length with regard to the Structural Futility Objection, human engineering of nature is now, for better or worse, a scientific given. It can hardly be denied, for instance, that many harmful interventions in nature have proven themselves successful. There are no good reasons to think differently when it comes to beneficial ones. Past and present experiences provide enough evidence for the increasing manageability of the alleged fixed laws of nature. Borrowing again from Gheaus, it may be noted that

> When tempted to declare things impossible in principle it is good to remember that we have already developed technologies allowing us to go against what people once believed were the laws of physics we can fly, or of biology we can cut open living bodies, extract functioning organs from them, sew them back, and find them still alive and well![22]

---

[16] Gheaus (2013, p. 455).   [17] *Ibid*, p. 449.
[18] See Gilabert (2012) for a distinction between soft and hard constraints.
[19] For a defense of this type of intervention, see Johannsen (2017, 2020).
[20] Pioneered by Pearce (2015 [2009]).   [21] For an overview, see Colyvan and Ginzburg (2003).
[22] Gheaus (2013, p. 455).

Animal Advocacy

Another way to increase the tractability of this cause is by putting wild animal suffering at the center of animal advocacy, that is, to raise awareness of wild animal suffering and its importance, as well as to encourage research in welfare biology in our daily activism. Some might say, however, that if what we should do is in general limited by what is possible to achieve, this is particularly true with regard to (animal) advocacy, where there is a higher expectation of short-term return.

As previously stated, there is a strong case for pushing further the limits of what is presently possible to achieve, though it is also the case, at least partially, that a substantial number of animal advocates are seemingly driven by short-term feasible goals (often referred to as "practical" or "pragmatic"). But this should not mean that the pursuit of short-term feasible goals should continue being one of the driving forces in promoting animal interests. In fact, as it has been reported by different organizations, traditional animal advocacy is highly cost-ineffective and subjected to many different biases. As an example, despite the fact that an overwhelming 99.6% of domesticated land animals used and killed by humans in the United States are farmed land animals, about 66% of donations to animal charities in the United States go to animal shelters.[23] To be sure, the responsibility of this cannot fully be attributed to animal advocacy, though it certainly suggests a clear margin for improvement.

Now, even if a certain level of concern with the feasibility or practicality of advocacy goals is recommended, it should always factor in the dynamic nature of what counts as feasible or practical across time.[24] This is not as controversial as it might at first seem. As a matter of fact, an increasingly crowded sector of animal activism is now focused on generating the circumstances that will make it increasingly feasible or practical to eradicate animal farming by investing resources on alternative methods of food production.

Thus, for all those interested in making effective animal activism part of their lives, a future-directed approach to advocacy should be preferred over a present-directed one. This is because in light of scientific and technological progress, the future holds the best opportunities for remedy of present harms, especially with regard to wild animal suffering. Given that the number of wild animals is largely predominant on the planet, we

---

[23] Animal Charity Evaluators (2016b).
[24] On the dynamic processes of political change, see Gilbert (2012).

should commit to maximizing future gains instead of sticking to presently feasible goals. This means acting now so as to make it possible that future people bring about the best states of affairs for wild animals.

Certainly, future people may be in a better position to address wild animal suffering and still fail to do so. This might be, for instance, because they ignore basic facts about wild animals' lives. This is why it is crucial that animal advocacy include raising awareness about how animals fare in the wild, by showing the evidence that counters the idyllic view of nature. Yet facts are usually not enough. People seem to act against X to the extent to which they know enough about X but also to the extent to which they care enough about X. This is why it is also necessary that animal advocacy include spreading the reasons for moral concern about wild animal suffering.

Spreading concern for wild animals now is of high expected value, especially considering future decision-making. The higher the concern for wild animal suffering among people, especially scientists and other experts, the more likely it will be, for instance, that wild animal–friendly environmental policies be undertaken.

To conclude, wild animal suffering is not intractable, nor interventions to reduce it are infeasible. To label certain interventions to reduce wild animal suffering as infeasible is merely to state that we cannot achieve them given our current state of knowledge. This is at best, only partially true, considering feasible low-impact interventions presently available. In addition, feasibility should be understood dynamically and conditional upon trying. With regard to large-scale interventions, we can affect their feasibility by putting ourselves in position to achieve them, both individually and collectively. This could mainly be done by developing welfare biology as a new field of research as well as by adopting a future-focused approach to animal advocacy. In sum, we can, and should, increase the tractability of wild animal suffering by working on its present neglectedness. The more people working on this issue, the more likely it is that safe and effective solutions to the plight of wild animals will be developed in the future.

Conclusion

It is commonly believed that our obligations toward other human beings are not restricted to abstaining from harming them. We should also prevent or alleviate harmful states of affairs for other individuals whenever it is in our power to do something about it. In animal ethics, however, the idea that we may have reasons not only to refrain from harming animals but also to help them is not particularly widespread. Of course, exceptions can be found regarding companion animals. Most people agree that failing to assist them would be wrong if we could otherwise help them. Most people give their companion animals veterinary care and believe such care should be extended to all captive animals. But what about all other animals in need, shouldn't we also help them? Consider *The Drowning Chimp* case introduced at the beginning of this book. Do you have an obligation to save the chimp? Consider also the numerous rescues of animals trapped in the ice or the recent efforts of Australian authorities and communities to help kangaroos, camels, horses, koalas, alpacas, and many other animals caught in the flames to survive as well as the aerial distribution of food in the days following the fires. Isn't that something that we ought to do?

It is sometimes claimed that even though interventions like this seem beneficial, the best we can do for animals living in nature is simply to let them be. In other words, we don't have reasons to prevent or alleviate the harms that animals suffer in the wild. This has been referred to as the "laissez-faire" intuition. This intuition usually relies on two fundamental assumptions. First, it is based on an idyllic view of nature, according to which wild animals have generally good lives, only threatened by occasional human interferences. Second, it is based on the idea that we only have reasons to help others in need when their situation is caused by human action. Nevertheless, there are compelling reasons to think that these two ideas are not justified.

First, contrary to what is often thought to be the case, animals living in the wild are subject to an enormous variety of threats to their well-being. They are usually injured, starved, or dehydrated. They must endure extreme weather conditions and cope with psychological stress, mainly due to fear of predation. They also experience excruciating deaths at the claws of predators, are devoured by parasites, and are debilitated or killed by disease. Moreover, this does not happen only to a few. The majority of wild animals follow a reproductive strategy that consists in increasing the population's fitness through the maximization of the number of offspring. The outcome of this is an extremely low survival rate. Most of the animals that come into existence do not survive to adulthood and have gruesome, short lives. This implies that most wild animals likely experience more suffering than positive well-being in their lives. Hence, on aggregate, suffering is likely to predominate in the wild. The idyllic view of nature is false, failing to provide grounds on which to base the *laissez-faire intuition*.

Second, *if* we think that positive moral obligations are generated by the relations of causality of harm, then what reasons may we have to help, say, a starving, distant, cognitively diverse human child[1]? We have not brought them into existence. We are not causally linked to the situation of vulnerability and dependence in which they encounter themselves. In addition, the child, given their severe cognitive disability, cannot recipro-cate and will never be able to do so. The harm they experience is a natural accident. In addition, we may suppose that they are a member of an isolated community of human beings. Nothing about their situation of need has been caused by the structures of domination and global inequal-ities through which humans have rendered other humans vulnerable. If, regardless, we believe that we ought to assist this child, then there must be different grounds for our positive duties of assistance. I claim that such is the case with the child's well-being. It is the value of the well-being of

---

[1] Notice that I am not endorsing a model of moral considerability according to which such a child would fall under the label of "marginal case," often used by mainstream animal ethicists. I believe that we should reject the very idea of marginal cases altogether. As Donaldson and Kymlicka have pointed out, "neurotypical human adults should never have been defined as the norm from which others are measured" (Donaldson and Kymlicka 2016, p. 239). I am aware though that the term "severe cognitive disability" may be perceived as lacking in specificity. I believe it is in the interest of this discussion to preserve a certain degree of generality so as to make the moral point of the example completely independent from the contingent, actual existence of certain (severe) cognitive disabilities. Although the appropriateness of the term bears little relevance to the substantive discussion, the example is still open to being criticized as a "vague hypothetical" (Taylor 2017, p. 131). I don't presently have definite solution to this problem.

sentient individuals, rather than how we relate to them, that generates positive obligations to help them.

Certainly, the capacity for well-being is not a phenomenon restricted to human children, but rather being exemplified by most nonhuman animals, including those living in the wild. Most people agree (at least, to some extent) that the well-being of animals (domesticated or wild) is what generates the negative duty to abstain from harming them. But if well-being imposes restrictions on what we may do to animals so as not to frustrate their interests, then well-being is also relevant to decide what we should do in order to actively promote the satisfaction of their interests. If the fact that animals can suffer is what generates the obligation to abstain from causing them to suffer, then that suffering is morally relevant no matter who or what causes it. Therefore, we should act in order to relieve it, whenever we can.

Some people might claim that there is a fundamental difference between human beings and domesticated animals, on the one hand, and animals that live in the wild, on the other, based on the former being "to a significant extent dependent on human beings' assistance," whereas the latter are not. Yet, there is no such difference. As facts about existence in the wild make apparent, animals that live there fare very poorly. As individuals, they lack the skills that would enable them to confront the harms posed by the environment and by other animals in a way that allows them to lead long, worthwhile lives. On the contrary, their lives are short and full of suffering. If there is anyone dependent on the assistance of human beings to avoid suffering and death, those are wild animals. If being dependent on human assistance is a source of positive obligations to assist those in need, animals in the wild qualify at least as much as humans and domesticated animals.

In a nutshell, this book argues that on the assumption that we have reasons to assist other individuals in need, there are decisive reasons to intervene in nature to prevent or reduce the harms wild animals suffer, provided that it is feasible and that the expected result is net positive.

In this book I claimed that *we have decisive reasons to prevent or reduce the harms wild animals suffer*. This conclusion relies on the following premises:

(1)   *Nonhuman animals are morally considerable (Chapter 1).*

Chapter 1 starts assuming the widespread view that having a well-being is necessary and sufficient for moral considerability. I then claimed that, on this view, nonhuman animals are morally considerable. This is because, insofar as they possess the capacity for conscious experiences, they have a

well-being of their own. After assuming this account of moral considerability, I assessed the objection that being sentient is not sufficient for
having a well-being. I concluded that under any plausible account of well-
being (hedonism, the desire-based view, or the objective-list theory), all
sentient individuals have a well-being of their own. Hence, nonhuman
animals are indeed morally considerable.

I then go on to evaluate the extent to which nonhuman well-being may
matter. To that end, I examined a widely employed principle in normative
ethics, namely, the principle of equal consideration of interests, according
to which equal interests count the same for moral purposes. If this
principle is correct, the claim that human interests in not suffering provide
us with stronger reasons to prevent their frustration than similar interests
in not suffering of nonhuman individuals is false.

In this chapter, I also disputed the widespread view that animals lack an
interest in being alive or, at most, that the strength of such interest is
always comparatively weaker than that of human beings. Given the divergence of competing views on this debate, my conclusions are conditional
in this regard. If death harms human beings for such and such reasons,
then, under the same assumptions, there are many nonhuman animals that
are also harmed by ceasing to exist. This allows, of course, for the
possibility that often the interest of a human being in continuing to live
may be stronger than the interest of a nonhuman animal. Nevertheless, the
opposite may also obtain. Animals can have, *in principle*, a stronger interest
in continued life than paradigmatic adults, even if, *in practice*, that might
not be common. Therefore, when discussing the badness of death, we
must reject the view that human and nonhuman animals harbor fundamentally different interests in being alive so that only humans benefit from
continued existence. Instead, if such interest exists, its strength simply
varies among individuals across species.

The discussion about the badness of death for nonhuman animals is
secondarily relevant in the context of intervention. If death (and not only
suffering) harms nonhuman animals, we thus have additional reasons to
act on their behalf, by preventing them from dying. At any rate, if ceasing
to exist does not harm sentient individuals at all (human and nonhuman),
we would still have reasons to act on their behalf by preventing or
otherwise reducing their suffering.

(2) *Speciesism is unjustified* (Chapter 2).

The previous conclusions may be disputed if speciesism is a justified moral
position. Given that the use of "speciesism" is usually ambiguous, in

Chapter 2 I examined the concept of speciesism by committing myself to an ameliorative inquiry. Accordingly, when engaging in antispeciesist theory, "speciesism" should be reserved for the unjustified instances of disadvantageous consideration or treatment of individuals that have the property of belonging to a certain species. I suggested, on the Wide Definition, that a certain position is speciesist if, and only if, it allows for the unjustified disadvantageous consideration or treatment of certain individuals, either by appeal to species membership alone or to criteria allegedly satisfied by the members of a certain species, and only by them. I thus rejected the Narrow Definition, which only classifies as speciesist positions that appeal to species membership.

There are several objections that can be presented against my proposed definition. First, according to the Overspeciesism Objection, this definition is overinclusive, insofar as it classifies as speciesist positions we would not normally classify as such. However, the charge of overspeciesism against the Wide Definition cannot succeed since the alternative Narrow Definition is clearly under-inclusive and would commit us to accepting as nonspeciesist positions that are definitely speciesist.

Next, I deal with the objection that speciesism is justified because anthropocentrism is. I show this stems from a confusion between speciesism and anthropocentrism. First, I disputed the claim that they are equivalent notions, and, second, the claim that anthropocentrism, because it is inevitable, justifies speciesism. Finally, I argued that moral anthropocentrism is unjustified and that it is indeed an instance of speciesism. This is shown by appeal to the argument from *species overlap* and the argument from relevance. These arguments can be used to show how no anthropocentric or non-anthropocentric appeal to species-specific attributes can justify the disadvantageous consideration of an individual.

I then argued for a categorical understanding of the concept of speciesism, instead of a gradual one. A certain speciesist position may vary according to the level of moral considerability it ascribes to animals, but that does not alter the fact that it is still an unjustified position. Therefore, there are no grounds for the claim that a position can be more or less speciesist. A position is either speciesist or not.

Finally, I examined a position that might be construed as a further instance of speciesism: Shelly Kagan's modal personism. According to this view, the interests of individuals who are either actual persons or could have been persons (modal persons) count more than the like interests of other nonperson individuals. I concluded that even if this position were right in identifying the modal property of being a person as morally relevant, it would still not allow for a justified moral distinction between individuals based on species membership. In addition, I argued that the property of being an actual person is irrelevant for the purposes of moral considerability and that, therefore, the property of being a modal person is so also irrelevant.

(3) *Suffering likely outweighs well-being in nature* (Chapter 3).

Taking similar human and nonhuman interests equally into account may require different courses of action from moral agents. It may often require that we refrain from harming nonhuman animals. On other occasions, it may demand that we benefit (or help) them whenever they are in a situation of need. This includes, of course, animals living in the wild. If wild animals had happy lives, intervening on their behalf would not be a highly important task. Nevertheless, far from it being a source of well-being for animals, evidence suggests that nature is rather a source of intense misery.

First, data from population dynamics tells us that due to the wasteful reproductive strategy favored by the majority of wild animals, suffering is largely present in nature. During their lives, wild animals are subjected to an enormous variety of natural threats to their health and physical integrity, which entails a great amount of suffering. They are usually injured, starved, or dehydrated. They must endure extreme weather conditions and cope with psychological stress, mainly due to fear of predation. In addition, wild animals experience excruciating deaths at the claws of predators, are harmed or devoured by parasites, and are debilitated or killed by disease. In light of such evidence, I concluded that we have strong reasons to intervene in nature in order to prevent or reduce wild animal suffering.

(4) *Perversity and futility objections against intervention fail* (Chapter 4).

Yet several objections may be put forward against the conclusion that intervening in nature is what we have most reason to do. In order to assess them, I first elaborated on Albert O. Hirschman's map of the rhetoric of reaction (perversity, futility, and jeopardy), which identifies the main theses of conservatism in its opposition to social change, and showed that a similar structure could be found in the narratives against intervention in nature. I further added three categories to that taxonomy: relationality, and tractability. Moreover, I distinguished those positions that agree that we have *decisive* reasons not to intervene in nature (perversity, futility, jeopardy, tractability, and Donaldson and Kymlicka's version of relationality) from those that believe that our reasons not to intervene are merely *sufficient* (Palmer's version of relationality).

Next, I considered the first set of objections – perversity and futility – that might be put forward against intervention in nature on behalf of wild animals. According to perversity objections, we should refrain from intervening because intervention will actually make things worse. According to futility objections, intervention should not be attempted because it is bound to fail. It will not be able to improve wild animal well-being, either due to structural (we cannot alter the basic structures of nature) or substantive (we cannot significantly increase wild animal well-being) limitations or because of feasibility (we cannot currently have an impact on wild animal well-being) concerns.

Then I assessed these objections. To that end, I subjected the arguments to Bostrom and Ord's *Reversal Test* and identified instances of status quo biases in them. I also provided additional reasons to reject these objections, when necessary. I concluded that no such objection succeeds in its defense of the claim that we have decisive reasons to oppose intervention. At most, these objections suggest what the interventionist may easily concede: That intervention, when feasible, should be performed just in case it is informed and when the expected outcome is net positive for wild animals.

(5) *Jeopardy objections to intervention fail* (Chapter 5).

In Chapter 5, I examined jeopardy objections, according to which intervention in nature should be prevented, insofar as it will threaten other, more important values. Depending on the theory endorsed, these values may vary. According to holistic views, these are values promoted either by the preservation of ecosystems (as suggested by ecocentrism) or the preservation of species taken as a whole (as in species holism). According to biocentric views, those values obtain through the preservation of other living entities such as plants and other non-sentient organisms. Finally, other views identify the "natural" and "the wilderness" as values to be preserved.

I assessed the cogency of these objections. I started by identifying several problems with holistic views. I argued that they either rely on an irrational preference for the status quo (thus failing at the *Reversal Test*) or build their case on implausible axiological assumptions, which lead to unacceptable consequences for the consideration of human interests. In addition, their value assessments regarding the preservation of ecological wholes (either ecosystems or species) are conditional on their impact on human well-being. Given that human and nonhuman interests should be given equal weight, the double-standard holistic opposition to intervention is unjustified. Moreover, they lack grounds on which to oppose all kinds of interventions to help animals, that is, to all those that do not tamper with holistic values.

I then examined the extent to which biocentric views offer a more compelling case against intervention. Yet I observed that such positions rely on a defective axiology and, when consistent, have implausible results. Moreover, it might be argued that rather than implying a rejection of helping wild animals in need actually supports it as part of a more general case to benefit all living things. Finally, I argued that the so-called "natural," understood as the result of evolution or as the natural wilderness, is revealed, at most, as possessing a kind of value that can be easily outweighed by that of nonhuman well-being and do not in any case imply an opposition to helping wild animals across the board. I thus concluded that intervention in nature on behalf of wild animals could not be opposed on jeopardy grounds. I finish the chapter with some remarks about pluralist accounts.

(6) *Relationality objections to intervention fail (Chapter 6).*

I then examined what we may term *relationality* objections to intervention in nature. These considerations have been advanced first and foremost by Clare Palmer and by Sue Donaldson and Will Kymlicka. I assessed and rejected Palmer's contextual account of our moral obligations toward animals in the wild. I started by reconstructing Palmer's view, according to which we have sufficient reasons not to intervene in nature. In particular, we are not usually required to assist wild animals due to the lack of prior morally relevant entanglements with them. I offered arguments for rejecting such relational considerations as grounds for determining the existence of positive moral obligations toward animals in the wild. Crucially, I claimed that, on any sound understanding of the view, it implausibly implies that there is no requirement to help *distant* human beings in need due to natural causes or to benefit other individuals even when that comes at no cost for the agent.

Next, I presented Donaldson and Kymlicka's view. I offered a strong case for construing Donaldson and Kymlicka's account in a way that implies that much more pervasive interventions in nature may be required – what I called *environmental enhancement*. Even if we have a duty to ensure that the environment provides for the satisfaction of wild animals' needs (as claimed by Donaldson and Kymlicka), facts suggest (Chapter 3) how the satisfaction of wild animals' interests does not depend, as these authors believe, on the preservation of their natural environments. Contrariwise, on this view, there would be a requirement to modify natural environmental conditions in a way that produces a net positive effect on nonhuman well-being.

Finally, I addressed some objections that might be put forward against this claim (fundamentally, replies grounded on considerations about flourishing) and concluded that appeals to relationality do not constitute sound objections against intervening in nature, especially in light of the magnitude of the harms experienced by wild animals.

(7)   *Priority objections to intervention fail* (Chapter 7).

I discussed different priority arguments against intervention in nature. They all share the idea that intervening to benefit wild animals should not be favored over benefiting human beings because that is what would bring about more value. The arguments put forward in support of this view may be systematized under three main approaches. First, on *the Exclusion Approach*, despite the very low levels of wild animal well-being, intervention is not a priority insofar as wild animals fall outside the scope of distributive principles (equality and priority). Most humans, however, are within such scope. Second, on *the Deflation Approach*, since nonhuman animals have a lower capacity for well-being (and a corresponding lower moral standing), increasing wild animal well-being produces less value than increasing the well-being of humans. Intervention in nature is, thus, not a priority. Finally, on *the Perfectionist Approach*, we should not intervene in nature for the sake of nonhuman animals because increases in nonhuman well-being cannot compensate for the loss of "the best things in life," only attainable by human activity. We should, thus, give priority to such increases in human well-being that ensure the existence of those excellent goods.

After assessing each of these approaches, I concluded that they face significant problems. Regarding the first two, they imply that the strength of equality and priority-based reasons varies even among rational agents, depending on the sophistication of their cognitive capacities. In addition, the problem cannot be solved by retreating to a threshold view since all such boundaries ultimately prove arbitrary. Furthermore, all three approaches have, additionally, highly unacceptable results. This can be particularly observed when considering scenarios that involve net negative levels of well-being. When faced with such scenarios, it seems implausible that our reasons to prefer other courses of action over preventing or alleviating great suffering are stronger. But the situation of wild animals in nature is indeed one such case. So, the same considerations should apply when those affected are nonhuman individuals. I, thus, concluded that priority objections also fail to provide us with decisive reasons not to prevent or alleviate the harms wild animals suffer.

Finally, I assessed the *Domesticated Animals First* objection, according to which while animal welfare is of salient moral concern, priority should be given to alleviating the harms suffered by domesticated animals, especially farmed animals. I claimed that either taken as a substantive or strategic objection, it cannot soundly succeed.

(8) *Tractability objections fail (Chapter 8).*

Wild animal suffering is not intractable, nor interventions to reduce it are infeasible. To label certain interventions to reduce wild animal suffering as infeasible is merely to state that we cannot achieve them given our current state of knowledge. This is, at best, only partially true, considering feasible low-impact interventions presently available. Beneficial interventions in nature already take place. In addition to occasional rescues, such as the one in our initial case, there are other, more significant ways in which we are already helping animals. Vaccination programs for wild animals against diseases such as rabies or tuberculosis have been implemented for decades. In national parks, starving animals are sometimes provided with additional food so that they may survive. These are just some examples among many. The success of these interventions suggests that many others would definitely be feasible as well. At any rate, the fundamental discussion is not about which ways of helping animals in nature are already available, but rather whether we have reasons to develop the means that will make it increasingly more feasible to help them. Feasibility should be understood dynamically and conditional upon trying. With regard to large-scale interventions, we can affect their feasibility by putting ourselves in a position to achieve them, both individually and collectively. This could mainly be done by developing welfare biology as a new field of research as well as by adopting a future-focused approach to animal advocacy.

Therefore, in light of the examination carried out in these eight chapters, we can conclude that the claim that we have decisive reasons to prevent or reduce the harms wild animals suffer stands.

* * *

In this book, I carried out an analysis of our reasons to prevent or reduce wild animal suffering. In the introduction, I claimed that the minimal case for intervention does not depend on assuming a particular normative position. Instead, it is premised on generally intuitive moral claims that many will find plausible, irrespective of their preferred normative theory. The first claim is, as stated, that we ought to aim at preventing or reducing the harms suffered by other individuals whenever it is in our power to do so. For short, we should help others whenever we can. This is something that can be accepted by a wide variety of moral theories. Consequentialists, for instance, will find it persuasive. All things being equal, helping others in need will bring about the greatest amount of good. For instance, it will maximize overall happiness. Non-consequentialists may also accept this basic claim. Deontologists may think we have, a least, a prima facie moral duty of beneficence, that is, a duty to do good to others, unless that duty is overridden by stronger moral considerations. Right theorists may also accept this insofar as they believe individuals have positive rights, including the right to receive assistance under certain circumstances. Accordingly, under such circumstances, we would have a duty provide the required assistance. Plausibly, virtue theorists would also accept that the sort of person we should become exhibits compassionate dispositions to act in the aforementioned way, that is, a character that exhibits the key virtues of compassion or kindness.

Regarding the second claim, on the moral considerability of nonhuman animals, it has been convincingly defended from a variety of moral theories, including utilitarianism,[2] egalitarianism,[3] rights theories,[4] contractualism,[5] Kantism,[6] the capabilities approach,[7] virtue ethics,[8] and care ethics,[9] just to name the most representative frameworks. It is not my place to rehearse their arguments here. We can confidently say that whatever normative theory one may endorse there will be sound reasons to believe that animal suffering matters. If that is so and suffering occurs in the lives of wild animals in numerous manners and often dramatically, we have strong reasons to intervene in nature so as to prevent or reduce that suffering whenever it is in our power to do so. In the end, the only bone of contention is whether those reasons are decisive. I hope this book has made a compelling case for the view that, indeed, they are.

---

[2] See, for example, Singer (2011, [1979]); de Lazari-Radek and Singer (2014); Varner (2012); Matheny (2006).
[3] See, for example, Persson (1993); Holtug (2007); Horta (2014), Faria (2014).
[4] See, for example, Regan (2004 [1983]); Cochrane (2012, 2019); Milburn (2017); Pepper (2020).
[5] See, for example, Rowlands (1998 [2009]).
[6] See, for example, Franklin (2005); Korsgaard (2018).   [7] See, for example, Nussbaum (2006).
[8] See, for example, Hursthouse (2011).   [9] See, for example, Adams (1991); (Donovan 2006).

Though this discussion has not been completely absent from the debates in animal ethics (as explained in the introduction), it has seldom benefited from a profound, comprehensive treatment.[10] I believe that the work carried out throughout this book constitutes, in this respect, a relevant contribution to the field. In particular:

(a) It develops the implications that follow from rejecting speciesism and including nonhuman animals that live in the wild into the sphere of full moral consideration due to all sentient individuals. In the literature, these implications have been either almost fully ignored or based on an incomplete assessment of how wild animals fare in nature. This book extends the scope of such implications by taking into account all natural events with a negative impact on wild animal well-being.

(b) Relatedly, this book disputes the widespread idyllic view of nature. It does this (i) by elaborating on the argument for the predominance of suffering over well-being in nature and (ii) by offering a systematic analysis of the empirical evidence that supports it. It shows that by failing to acknowledge these facts, most authors have been deficient in their assessment of wild animal well-being. This is crucial, because even assuming for the sake of the argument that there might be reasons not to intervene in nature given by considerations different from the well-being of animals, the magnitude of wild animal suffering suggests that it is false that those reasons are sufficient.

(c) It develops a comprehensive taxonomy of the different objections that have been (or might be) put forward against intervention in nature. In the literature, these objections are usually presented in a scattered or indirect way. By elaborating on Albert O. Hirschman's map of the opposition to social progress (consisting of three main theses: perversity, futility, jeopardy), I suggest that the central case against intervention might be systematized as consisting of six main sets of objections: (i) perversity, (ii) futility, (iii) jeopardy, (iv) relationality, (v) priority, and (vi) tractability. The taxonomy also reveals the similarity between the anti-interventionist and the conservative discourses.

(d) Finally, it offers an assessment of each of these sets of objections against intervention in nature, some of which had not been previously addressed in the literature, providing new arguments against them.

---

[10] A salient counterexample to this unfortunate rule is Johannsen (2020).

There are, however, a number of relevant philosophical issues that this book could not cover. For example, just as many discussions on the priority that ought to be given to the worst off do not address the problem about interpersonal comparison of utility, I have not discussed interspecies comparisons of well-being. Neither have I addressed the structure of the good or whether it matters, in itself, how the good is distributed among individuals. For instance, it seems that our reasons to reduce, or eliminate, future wild animal suffering will be stronger according to egalitarian, prioritarian, or sufficientarian views. Therefore, in order to refine the conclusions of this book, more work needs to be done.

Second, this normative research ought to be complemented by further investigation about specific forms of feasible, effective, and net-positive interventions in nature to help animals at a small or medium scale. This is not, of course, a task for a philosopher. The fundamental discussion in this book could not be focused on which ways of helping animals in nature are already available, but rather on whether we have reasons to develop the means that will make it increasingly more feasible to help them in the future. Nevertheless, ecologists, animal welfare scientists, and other life scientists working on related issues can pursue such goals and help thus advance the largely neglected field of "welfare biology" – that is, the systematic research on how we can improve the well-being of wild animals.

Third, this research does not address the question of what would be the best political framework to carry out interventions in nature once the moral case is settled. Some implications have recently been explored though.[11] It has been suggested that the moral case implies a re-examination and expansion of the limits of our political communities such that membership is defined not in terms of the inherent worthiness of *homo sapiens*, but in terms of who is likely to be affected by human policy-making and institutional practices, thereby truly rejecting parochialism, whatever its form. As some cosmopolitans have recently stressed, "Such partiality leads us to unfairly prioritize some, while neglecting others; and it leads us to neglect of the fact that it is the sentient individual who is of ultimate moral worth, not the groups of which they are a part."[12] The question of how to effectively apply such a cosmopolitan interspecies is beyond the scope of this book. The main goal here is not to develop a non-speciesist political framework, but rather to provide the moral grounds to

[11] Cochrane (2018); Johannsen (2020).   [12] Cochrane (2018), p. 4.

sustain it, even if, at some points, the discussion (necessarily) overlaps with more political concerns.

Fourth, this book does not provide an assessment of the impact of current policies of environmental management on the well-being of animals. Consider, for instance, conservation programs of large herbivores, such as elephants, which have the potential to reduce the suffering of animals in the wild on aggregate. For instance, the presence of large herbivores has a high potential to reduce the overall levels of suffering within an ecosystem. If so, we should promote the expansion of these populations as an ethically effective measure of environmental management and ecosystem engineering. To inform these policies, however, much more research in welfare biology needs to be done.

Fifth, this research is relevant for current debates in population ethics. A complete and unbiased population axiology ought to be designed so as to rank populations that also include wild animals. Factoring in wild animal well-being will have important implications for assessments of environmental damage and global existential risks (specially s-risks[13]). If morally considerable entities are also nonhuman, to the extent that where we can affect those entities and processes not only present, but also future ones, we have reasons to follow those courses of action that are better from the point of view of what is best for such entities. Identifying these courses of action is not an easy task since it requires discussing the challenges posed by the problem of nonidentity.[14] Despite different attempts to solve this paradox,[15] the discussions are currently limited to scenarios involving exclusively human beings, excluding other sentient individuals from the discussion. It is therefore necessary to develop a framework for thinking about the future that responds to the challenges posed by the nonidentity problem that is not limited to consideration of future human generations. And if this is important in general, it seems particularly pressing in view of the urgency to develop a sound ethical framework that takes into account the increasing impact of climate change. On the other hand, it is possible that the response itself to climate change may bring about scenarios with astronomical amounts of suffering. As we have seen, a significant number

---

[13] A suffering-risk or s-risk is defined as "[o]ne where an adverse outcome would bring about severe suffering on an astronomical scale, vastly exceeding all suffering that has existed on Earth so far." Althaus and Gloor (2016). See also Sotala and Gloor (2017, p. 389).

[14] Parfit (1984).

[15] See, for example, Broome (1994), Boonin (2008), Singer (2011), Feldman (1992), Temkin (2012).

of animals who live in nature suffer greatly as a result of living in ecosystems in which predation, disease, and death premature are endemic. And there is a high risk that the current state of affairs be reproduced in the design of future sentient beings and ecosystems. For the time being, with the technology already available, programs to recreate natural ecosystems are already being implemented ("rewilding"), thereby plausibly amplifying existing suffering. This situation can be further magnified when future technology allows human beings, for example, to terraform other planets. Since terraforming would take place in a world insensitive to nonhuman suffering, it is highly probable that a terraformed planet would contain as much or more suffering as there is now on earth, thus multiplying suffering in the universe at an astronomical scale.[16]

Finally, this book does not deliberately engage with arguments from hubris, however common they may be, according to which, roughly, intervening in nature would somehow reflect an overconfidence on human capacities and therefore be fatally contaminated by anthropocentric bias in favor of "human values." I am sure there is a lot of relevant work that could be done to address this concern. Let me just briefly say that to recognize that suffering and death are bad is by no means a "human value." To claim that suffering and death are bad for those who experience it irrespective of their species entails precisely rejecting anthropocentrism and not the other way around. In addition, whether we want it or not, we (will) increasingly have the power to engineer the world around us. The question is then one of determining to what ends that power will be put to use. A plausible answer is that it should be placed at the service of the common good. Or so I hope to have convincingly argued.

Some might say that the conclusions reached throughout this book are, perhaps, too demanding. In reply, let me simply state I do not believe this is so. Rather, it is because the world is so far removed from the best possible scenario that such demands are made on us. Demandingness objections in general rely on the assumption that any moral theory that makes substantial requirements of us is, on its face, less plausible than a theory that does not. However, it is not clear why a low degree of demandingness should be considered a theoretical virtue in ethics. In fact,

---

[16] For a related discussion, see O'Brien, G. D. (2021).

the state of the world is so calamitous that any plausible moral theory must entail that hard sacrifices are required. As I mentioned in the first page of this book, we should be wary of *cosy* moral beliefs. Philosophers should be revisionists.[17] If our beliefs are wrong, we should change them. If things are bad, we should act accordingly.

[17] On the distinction between descriptive and revisionist philosophy, see Parfit (1984, preface).

References

Aaltola, E. (2008). Personhood and animals. *Environmental ethics, 30*(2), 175–193.

(2012). *Animal suffering: Philosophy and culture.* Palgrave MacMillan.

Abbott, D. H., Keverne, E. B., Bercovitch, F. B., Shively, C. A., Mendoza, S. P., Saltzman, W., ... Sapolsky, R. M. (2003). Are subordinates always stressed? A comparative analysis of rank differences in cortisol levels among primates. *Hormones and behavior, 43*(1), 67–82.

Academy of Achievement (2009, July 6). *Jane Goodall – Interview: The woman who redefined man.* www.achievement.org/autodoc/page/goo1int-3

Adam, R. A. (2011). Biology of *Giardia lambia. Clinical Microbiology Review, 14* (3), 447–475.

Adams, C. J. (1991). Ecofeminism and the eating of animals. *Hypatia, 6*(1), 125–145.

Adams, C. J., & Donovan, J. (Eds.) (1995). *Animals and women: Feminist theoretical explorations.* Duke University Press.

Agar, N. (1997). Biocentrism and the concept of life. *Ethics, 108*(1), 147–168.

Ahmed-Farid, O. A., Salah, A. S., Nassan, M. A., & El-Tarabany, M. S. (2021). Effects of chronic thermal stress on performance, energy metabolism, anti-oxidant activity, brain serotonin, and blood biochemical indices of broiler chickens. *Animals, 11*(9), 2554.

Albersmeier, F. (2021). Speciesism and speciescentrism. *Ethical Theory and Moral Practice, 24*(2), 511–527.

Allen, C., & Bekoff, M. (1997). *Species of mind: The philosophy and biology of cognitive ethology.* MIT Press.

Alonso, W. J., & Schuck-Paim, C. (2017). Life-fates: Meaningful categories to estimate animal suffering in the wild. *Animal Ethics.* www.animal-ethics.org/life-fates-essay-prize-2017

Althaus, D., & Gloor, L. (2016, September 14). Reducing risks of astronomical suffering: A neglected priority. *Foundational Research Institute.* https://foundational-research.org/reducing-risks-of-astronomical-suffering-a-neglected-priority/

American Psychological Association (2020). *Publication manual of the American Psychological Association* (8th ed.). American Psychological Association.

Anderson, J. C. (1993). Species equality and the foundations of moral theory. *Environmental Values*, 2(4), 347–365.

Anholt, B. R., & Werner, E. E. (1995). Interaction between food availability and predation mortality mediated by adaptive behavior. *Ecology*, 76(7), 2230–2234.

(1998). Predictable changes in predation mortality as a consequence of changes in food availability and predation risk. *Evolutionary Ecology*, 12(6), 729–738.

Animal Charity Evaluators (2016a). Does animal advocacy messaging influence support for policies affecting wild animal suffering? *Animal Charity Evaluators*. https://osf.io/jj23a/

(2016b). Why farmed animals? *Animal Charity Evaluators*. https://animalcha rityevaluators.org/donation-advice/why-farmed-animals/

Armstrong, S. J., & Botzler, R. G. (Eds.). (2003). *The animal ethics reader*. Routledge.

Arneson, R. (1999). What, if anything, renders all humans morally equal? In Jamieson, D. (Ed.), *Singer and his critics* (pp. 103–128). Blackwell.

(2000). Welfare should be the currency of justice. *Canadian Journal of Philosophy*, 30(4), 497–524.

(2014). Basic equality: Neither rejectable nor acceptable. In Steinhoff, U. (Ed.), *Do all persons have equal moral worth? On "basic equality" and equal respect and concern* (pp. 30–52). Oxford University Press.

Ashley, E. A., Olson, J. K., Adler, T. E., Raverty, S., Anderson, E. M., Jeffries, S., & Gaydos, J. K. (2020). Causes of mortality in a harbor seal (*Phoca vitulina*) population at equilibrium. *Frontiers in Marine Science*, 7, 319.

Attfield, R. (1983). *The ethics of environmental concern*. Basil Blackwell.

(1987). Biocentrism, moral standing and moral significance. *Philosophica*, 39, 47–58.

Australian Geographic (2012, July 3). Devil tumour disease a parasite, say experts. *Australian Geographic*. http://cms.ausgeo.bauer-media.net.au/news/2012/07/devil-tumour-disease-a-parasite,-say-experts

Bailey, R., Seymour, N., & Stewart, G. (1978). Rape behavior in blue-winged teal. *Short Communications*, 95, 188–190.

Balcombe, J. P. (2006). *Pleasurable kingdom: Animals and the nature of feeling good*. Macmillan.

Battin, J. (2004). When good animals love bad habitats: Ecological traps and the conservation of animal populations. *Conservation Biology*, 18(6), 1482–1491.

Becker, L. C. (1983). The priority of human interests. In Miller, H. B., & Williams, W. H. (Eds.), *Ethics and animals* (pp. 225–242). Humana Press.

Beer, J. V., & Ogilvie, M. A. (1972). Mortality. In Scott, P., & The Wildfowl Trust (Eds.), *The swans* (pp. 125–142). Houghton-Mifflin.

Bekoff, M. (2010). *The animal manifesto: Six reasons for expanding our compassion footprint*. New World Library.

(2013). *Ignoring nature no more*. The University of Chicago Press.

Belshaw, C. (2014 [2009]). *Annihilation: The sense and significance of death*. Routledge.

Benton, T. (1993). *Natural relations: Ecology, animal rights, and social justice.* Verso.

Berdoy, M., Webster, J. P., & Macdonald, D. W. (2000). Fatal attraction in rats infected with *Toxoplasma gondii. Proceedings of the Royal Society of London B: Biological Sciences, 267*(1452), 1591–1594.

Berger, L., Speare, R., Hines, H. B., Marantelli, G., Hyatt, A. D., McDonald, K. R., . . . Tyler, M. J. (2004). Effect of season and temperature on mortality in amphibians due to chytridiomycosis. *Australian Veterinary Journal, 82*(7), 434–439.

Bernstein, M. H. (1998). *On moral considerability: An essay on who morally matters.* Oxford University Press.

(2002). Marginal cases and moral relevance. *Journal of Social Philosophy, 33*(4), 523–539.

(2004). Neo-speciesism. *Journal of Social Philosophy, 35*(3), 380–390.

(2015). *The moral equality of humans and animals.* Palgrave MacMillan.

Bexton, S., & Robinson, I. (2003). Hedgehogs. In Mullineaux, E., Best, R., & Cooper, J. E. (Eds.), *BSAVA manual of wildlife casualties* (2nd ed., pp. 49–65). British Small Animal Veterinary Association.

Biggers, J. D., Finn, C. A., & McLaren, A. (1962). Long-term reproductive performance of female mice. *Journal of Reproduction and Fertility, 3*(3), 313–330.

Biknevicius, A. R., & Van Valkenburgh, B. (2019). Design for killing: Craniodental adaptations of predators. In Gittleman, J. L. (Ed.), *Carnivore behavior, ecology, and evolution* (pp. 393–428). Cornell University Press.

Biondi, M., & Zannino, L. G. (1997). Psychological stress, neuroimmunomodulation, and susceptibility to infectious diseases in animals and man: A review. *Psychotherapy and Psychosomatics, 66*(1), 3–26.

Birch, J. (2020). The search for invertebrate consciousness. *Noûs.* 1–21. https://doi.org/10.1111/nous.12351

Bleicher, S. S. (2017). The landscape of fear conceptual framework: Definition and review of current applications and misuses. *PeerJ, 5*(9), e3772.

Boonin, D. (2008). How to solve the non-identity problem. *Public Affairs Quarterly, 22*(2), 129–159.

Bostrom, N., & Ord, T. (2006). The reversal test: Eliminating status quo bias in applied ethics. *Ethics, 16*(4), 656–679.

Botreau, R., Veissier, I., Butterworth, A., Bracke, M. B., & Keeling, L. J. (2007). Definition of criteria for overall assessment of animal welfare. *Animal Welfare-Potters Bar Then Wheathampstead, 16*(2), 225.

Bovenkerk, B., Stafleu, F., Tramper, R., Vorstenbosch, J., & Brom, F. W. A. (2003). To act or not to act? Sheltering animals from the wild: A pluralistic account of a conflict between animal and environmental ethics. *Ethics, Place and Environment, 6*(1), 13–26.

Bowler, D. E., Haase, P., Hof, C., Kröncke, I., Baert, L., Dekoninck, W., . . . & Böhning-Gaese, K. (2017). Cross-taxa generalities in the relationship between population abundance and ambient temperatures. *Proceedings of the Royal Society B: Biological Sciences, 284*(1863), 20170870.

Boyd, B. S., Colon, F., Doty, J. F., & Sanders, K. C. (2021). Beware of the dragon: A case report of a komodo dragon attack. *Foot & Ankle Orthopaedics, 6*(2), 24730114211015623.

Bradley, B. (2009). *Well-being and death.* Oxford University Press.

Braithwaite, V. (2010). *Do fish feel pain?* Oxford University Press.

Bramble, B. (2021). Painlessly killing predators. *Journal of Applied Philosophy, 38* (2), 217–225.

Brennan, A. (1998). *Thinking about nature: An investigation of nature, value and ecology.* Routledge.

Bro-Jørgensen, J. (2013). Evolution of sprint speed in African savannah herbivores in relation to predation. *Evolution, 67*(11), 3371–3376.

Broad, C. D. (1938). *Examination of McTaggart's philosophy.* Cambridge University Press.

Broom, D. M., & Johnson, K. G. (1993). *Stress and animal welfare.* Kluwer.

Broome, J. (1994). Discounting the future. *Philosophy & Public Affairs, 23*(2), 128–156.

(2004). *Weighing lives.* Oxford University Press.

Broom, D. M. (2014). *Sentience and animal welfare.* CABI.

Brown, C. R., & Brown, M. B. (1998). Intense natural selection on body size and wing and tail asymmetry in cliff swallows during severe weather. *Evolution, 52*(5), 1461–1475.

Bruers, S. (2014). *Born free and equal? On the ethical consistency of animal equality.* Lambert Academic Publishing.

(2015). The core argument for veganism. *Philosophia, 43*(2), 271–290.

Buchanan, A. (2011). *Better than human: The promise and perils of enhancing ourselves.* Oxford University Press.

Buffalo Field Campaign (2016). Vaccination of wild buffalo fact sheet. www .buffalofieldcampaign.org/factsheets/bisonvaccinationfact.html.

Burghardt, G. M. (2013). Beyond suffering – commentary on Clare Palmer. *Between the Species, 16*(1), 5. http://digitalcommons.calpoly.edu/bts/vol16/iss1/5/.

Bush. M. (1986 [1985]). Laparoscopy and surgery. In Fowler, M. E. (Ed.), *Zoo and wild animal medicine* (pp. 253–261). WB Saunders & Co.

Callicott, J. B. (1980). Animal liberation: A triangular affair. *Environmental Ethics, 2*(4), 311–338.

(1988). Animal liberation and environmental ethics: Back together again, *Between the Species, 4*(3), 3, 163–169, http://digitalcommons.calpoly.edu/bts/vol4/iss3/3/.

(1989). *In defense of the land ethic: Essays in environmental philosophy.* State University of New York.

(2000). Contemporary criticism of the received wilderness idea. In Cole, D. N., McCool, S. F., Freimund, W. A., & O'Loughlin, J. (Comps.), *Wilderness science in a time of change conference. Volume 1: Changing perspectives and future directions* (pp. 23–27). U.S. Department of Agriculture, Forest Service, Rocky Mountain Research Station.

Callicott, J. B., & Nelson, M. P. (Eds.). (1998). *The great new wilderness debate.* University of Georgia Press.

Carlstead, K. Brown, J. L., & Strawn, W. (1993). Behavioral and physiological correlates of stress in laboratory cats. *Applied Animal Behaviour Science, 38* (2), 143–158.

Carpendale, M. (2015). Welfare biology as an extension of biology: Interview with Yew-Kwang Ng. *Relations: Beyond Anthropocentrism 3*(2), 197–202.

Carruthers, P. (1992). *The animal issue: Moral theory in practice.* Cambridge University Press.

Cavalieri, P. (2001). *The animal question: Why nonhuman animals deserve human rights.* Oxford University Press.

(2006). Ethics, animals and the nonhuman great apes. *Journal of Biosciences, 31* (5), 509–512.

Cavalieri, P., & Singer, P. (Eds.). (1993). *The Great Ape Project: Equality beyond humanity.* St. Martin's Press.

Chapman, C. A., Wasserman, M. D., Gillespie, T. R., Speirs, M. L., Lawes, M. J., Saj, T. L., & Ziegler, T. E. (2006). Do food availability, parasitism, and stress have synergistic effects on red colobus populations living in forest fragments?, *American Journal of Physical Anthropology, 131*(4), 525–534.

Cheney, J. (1989). Postmodern environmental ethics: Ethics as bioregional narrative. *Environmental Ethics, 11*(2), 117–134.

Chin, L., Moran, J. A., & Clarke, C. (2010). Trap geometry in three giant montane pitcher plant species from Borneo is a function of tree shrew body size. *New Phytologist, 186*(2), 461–470.

Cigman, R. (1980). Death, misfortune, and species inequality. *Philosophy and Public Affairs, 10*, 47–64.

Cirillo, D., & Valencia, A. (2018). Algorithmic complexity in Computational Biology. *arXiv preprint arXiv:1811.07312.*

Clark, S. R. L. (1977). *The moral status of animals.* Oxford University Press.

Clarke, C. M., Bauer, U., Ch'ien, C. L., Tuen, A. A., Rembold, K., & Moran, J. A. (2009). Tree shrew lavatories: A novel nitrogen sequestration strategy in a tropical pitcher plant. *Biology Letters, 5*(5), 632–635.

Clarke, M., & Ng, Y.-K. (2006). Population dynamics and animal welfare: Issues raised by the culling of kangaroos in Puckapunyal. *Social Choice and Welfare, 27*(2), 407–422.

Clement, G. (2003). The ethic of care and the problem of wild animals. *Between the Species*, 13(3), 1–12 http://digitalcommons.calpoly.edu/bts/vol13/iss3/2/.

Clinchy, M., Zanette, L., Boonstra, R., Wingfield, J. C., & Smith, J. N. M. (2004). Balancing food and predator pressure induces chronic stress in songbirds. *Proceedings of the Royal Society of London B: Biological Sciences, 271*(1556), 2473–2479.

Clubb, R., & Mason, G. (2003).Captivity effects on wide-ranging carnivores. *Nature, 425*(6957), 473–474.

Cochrane, A. (2012). *Animal rights without liberation*. Columbia University Press.
  (2013). Cosmozoopolis: The case against group-differentiated animal rights. *Law, Ethics and Philosophy, 1*, 127–41.
  (2018). *Sentientist politics: A theory of global inter-species justice*. Oxford University Press.
Coghlan, S., & Cardilini, A. P. (2021). A critical review of the compassionate conservation debate. *Conservation Biology*. 1–15. https://doi.org/10.1002/cobi.13760
Cohen, C. (1986). The case for the use of animals in biomedical research. *New England Journal of Medicine, 315*, 865–870.
Cohen, C., & Regan, T. (2001). *The animal rights debate*. Rowman & Littlefield.
Cohn, P. (Ed.). (1999). *Ethics and wildlife*. Edwin Mellen.
Cole, R. A., & Friend, M. (1999). Miscellaneous parasitic diseases. In Friend, M., & Franson, J. C. (Eds.), *Field manual of wildlife diseases: General field procedures and diseases of birds. Biological Resources Division Information and Technology Report 1999-001* (pp. 249–258). US Geological Survey.
Colyvan, M., & Ginzburg, L. R. (2003). Laws of nature and laws of ecology. *Oikos, 101*(3), 649–653.
Connor, R. C., Smolker, R. A., & Richards, A. F. (1992). Dolphin alliances and coalitions. In Harcourt, A. H., & de Waal, F. B. M. (Eds.), *Coalitions and alliances in humans and other animals* (pp. 415–442). Oxford University Press.
Conover, M. R., Dinkins, J. B., & Haney, M. J. (2013). Impacts of weather and accidents on wildlife. In Hopkins Press, *Wildlife management and conservation: Contemporary principles and practices* (pp. 144–155). Johns Hopkins University Press.
Corner, L. A. (2006). The role of wild animal populations in the epidemiology of tuberculosis in domestic animals: How to assess the risk. *Veterinary Microbiology, 112*(2-4), 303–312.
Cowen, T. (2003). Policing nature. *Environmental Ethics, 25*(2), 169–182.
Crisp, R. (1998). Animal liberation is not an environmental ethic: A response to Dale Jamieson. *Environmental Values, 7*(4), 476–478.
  (1994). Values, reasons, and the environment. In Belsey A., & Attfield R. (Eds.), *Philosophy and the natural environment* (pp. 75–87). Cambridge University Press.
Cruz-Flores, M., Pradel, R., Bried, J., González-Solís, J., & Ramos, R. (2021). Sex-specific costs of reproduction on survival in a long-lived seabird. *Biology Letters, 17*(3), 20200804.
Culina, A., Linton, D. M., Pradel, R., Bouwhuis, S., & Macdonald, D. W. (2019). Live fast, don't die young: Survival–reproduction trade-offs in long-lived income breeders. *Journal of Animal Ecology, 88*(5), 746–756.
Cunha, L. C. (2015). If natural entities have intrinsic value, should we then abstain from helping animals who are victims of natural processes. *Beyond Anthropocentrism, 3*, 51.

Cushing, S. (2003). Against 'humanism': Speciesism, personhood and preference. *Journal of Social Philosophy*, *34*(4), 556–571.

Dantzer, R., & Mormède, P. (1983). Stress in farm animals: A need for reevaluation, *Journal of Animal Science*, *57*(1), 6–18.

Darwin, C. (1856). Letter to J. D. Hooker. Darwin Project. University of Cambridge. www.darwinproject.ac.uk/letter/DCP-LETT-1924.xml

Dawkins, M. (2012 [1980]). *Animal suffering: The science of animal welfare.* Springer.

Dawkins, R. (1995). God's utility function. *Scientific American*, *273*(5), 80–85.

de Lazari-Radek, K., & Singer, P. (2014). *The point of view of the universe: Sidgwick and contemporary ethics.* Oxford University Press.

De Grazia, D. (1996). *Taking animals seriously: Mental life and moral status.* Cambridge University Press.

(1997). Great apes, dolphins and the concept of personhood. *Southern Journal of Philosophy*, *35*(3), 301–320.

(2016) Modal personhood and moral status: A reply to Kagan's proposal. *Journal of Applied Philosophy*, *33*(1), 22–25.

Delahay, R. J., Smith, G. C., & Hutchings, M. R. (2009) *Management of disease in wild mammals.* Springer.

DelGiudice, G. D., Riggs, M. R., Joly, P., & Pan, W. (2002). Winter severity, survival, and cause-specific mortality of female white-tailed deer in North-Central Minnesota. *Journal of Wildlife Management*, *66*, 698–717.

Dell'Amore, C. (2010, July 15). Despite 'poor imitation,' cat shows surprising 'psychological cunning'. *National Geographic News* http://news.nationalgeographic.com/news/2010/07/100712-cats-mimics-monkeys-prey-science/.

Delmas, C. (2014a). Samaritanism and political legitimacy. *Analysis*, *74*(2), 254–262.

(2014b). Samaritanism and civil disobedience. *Res Publica*, *20*(3), 295–313.

Delon, N., & Purves, D. (2018). Wild animal suffering is intractable. *Journal of Agricultural and Environmental Ethics*, *31*(2), 239–260.

Diamond, C. (1978). Eating meat and eating people. *Philosophy* *53*(206), 465–479.

(1991). The importance of being human. *Royal Institute of Philosophy Supplements*, *29*, 35–62.

Dias, P. C. (1996). Sources and sinks in population biology. *Trends in Ecology and Evolution*, *11*(8), 326–330.

Díaz-León, E. (2020). Descriptive vs. Ameliorative Projects: The role of normative considerations. In Burgess, A., Cappelen, H., & D. Plunkett (Eds.), *Conceptual engineering and conceptual ethics* (pp. 170–186). Oxford University Press.

Dickens, M. J., Earle, K. A., & Romero, L. M. (2009). Initial transference of wild birds to captivity alters stress physiology. *General and Comparative Endocrinology*, *160* (1), 76–83.

Dixon, B. R., Parenteau, M., Martineau, C., & Fournier, J. (1997). A comparison of conventional microscopy, immunofluorescence microscopy and flow cytometry in the detection of Giardia lamblia cysts in beaver fecal samples. *Journal of Immunological Methods, 202*(1), 27–33.

Dobson, F. S., & Jouventin, P. (2010). The trade-off of reproduction and survival in slow-breeding seabirds. *Canadian Journal of Zoology, 88*(9), 889–899.

Dombrowski, D. A. (1996). *Babies and beasts: The argument from marginal cases.* University of Illinois Press.

(2006). Is the argument from marginal cases obtuse? *Journal of Applied Philosophy, 23*(2), 223–232.

Donaldson, S., & Kymlicka, W. (2011a) *Zoopolis: A political theory of animal rights.* Oxford University Press.

(2011b). *Zoopolis: A political theory of animal rights*: An overview. *Academia.edu,* www.academia.edu/2394382/Sue_Donaldson_and_Will_Kymlicka_Zoopo lis_A_Political_Theory_of_Animal_Rights_An_Overview_.

(2013). A defense of animal citizens and sovereigns. *Law, Ethics and Philosophy, 1,* 143–160.

Donaldson, S., & Kymlicka, W. (2016). Rethinking membership and participation in an inclusive democracy: Cognitive disability, children, animals. *Disability and political theory,* 168–197.

Donovan, J. (2006). Feminism and the treatment of animals: From care to dialogue. *Signs: Journal of Women in Culture and Society, 31*(2), 305–329.

Donovan, J., & Adams, C. J. (Eds.). (1996). *Beyond animal rights: A feminist caring ethic for the treatment of animals.* Continuum.

Donovan, J., & Adams, C. J. (Eds.). (2007). *The feminist care tradition in animal ethics: A reader.* Columbia University Press.

Dorado, D. (2015). Ethical interventions in the wild. An annotated bibliography. *Relations: Beyond Anthropocentrism, 3*(1), 219–238.

Du Toit, J. G. (2001). *Veterinary care of African elephants.* Novartis & South African Veterinary Foundation.

Dunayer, J. (2004). *Speciesism.* Ryce.

Dworkin, R. (1993). *Life's dominion: An argument about abortion and euthanasia.* Harper Collins.

Ebert, R., & Machan, T. R. (2012). Innocent threats and the problem of carnivorous animals. *Journal of Applied Philosophy, 29*(2), 146–159.

Ehnert, J. (2002). The argument from species overlap, MA thesis, Blacksburg: Virginia Polytechnic Institute and State.

Elliot, R. (1997). *Faking nature: The ethics of environmental restoration.* Routledge.

Epicurus (1964 [ca. 300 BC]). *Letter to Menoeceus,* in his *Letters, principal doctrines and Vatican sayings.* Bobbs-Merrill, 53–59.

Erman, E., & Möller, N. (2020). A world of possibilities: The place of feasibility in political theory. *Res Publica, 26*(1), 1–23.

Evans, G. H. (1910). *Elephants and their diseases: A treatise on elephants.* Government Printing.

Evans, H. C., Elliot, S. L., & Hughes, D. P. (2011). Hidden diversity behind the zombie-ant fungus Ophiocordyceps unilateralis: Four new species described from carpenter ants in Minas Gerais, Brazil. *PloS One, 6*(3), e17024.

Everett, J. (2001). Environmental ethics, animal welfarism, and the problem of predation: A bambi lover's respect for nature. *Ethics and the Environment*, 6, 42–67.

FAO – Food and Agriculture Organization of the United Nations (2019) "Livestock primary", *FAO statistical database*, http://www.fao.org/faostat/en/#data/QCL

Faria, C. (2011). Pessoas não humanas: A consideração moral dos grandes símios e outras criaturas. *Diacrítica*, 25, 33–50.

(2013). Differential obligations towards others in need. *Astrolabio*, 15, 242–246.

(2014). Equality, priority and nonhuman animals. *Dilemata*, 14, 225–236.

(2015). Making a difference on behalf of animals living in the wild: Interview with Jeff McMahan. *Relations: Beyond Anthropocentrism*, 3(1), 81–84.

(2016). Why we should not postpone awareness of wild animal suffering. *Animal Sentience*, 1(7), 14.

Faria, C., & Horta, O. (2019). Welfare biology. In Taylor and Francis Group, *The Routledge Handbook of Animal Ethics* (pp. 455–466). Routledge.

Faria, C., & Paez, E. (2015). Animals in need: The problem of wild animal suffering and intervention in nature. *Relations: Beyond Anthropocentrism*, 3 (1), 7–13.

(2014). Anthropocentrism and speciesism: Conceptual and normative issues. *Rev. Bioetica & Derecho*, 32, 95.

(2019). It's Splitsville: Why animal ethics and environmental ethics are incompatible. *American Behavioral Scientist*, 63(8), 1047–1060.

Fehige, C. (1998). A Pareto principle for possible people. In Fehige, C., & Wessels, U. (Eds.), *Preferences* (pp. 508–543). de Gruyter.

Feinberg, J. (1980). The rights of animals and unborn generations. In The University Press Group, *Rights, Justice, and the Bounds of Liberty. Essays in social philosophy* (pp. 159–184). Princeton University Press.

Feit, N. (2002). The time of death's misfortune. *Noûs*, 36(3), 359–383.

Feldman, F. (1992). *Confrontations with the reaper: A philosophical study of the nature and value of death*. Oxford University Press.

(1995). Justice, desert, and the repugnant conclusion. *Utilitas*, 7(2), 567–585.

(2004). *Pleasure and the good life*. Oxford University Press.

Ferdowsian, H., & Merskin, D. (2012). Parallels in sources of trauma, pain, distress, and suffering in humans and nonhuman animals. *Journal Trauma Dissociation*, 3(4), 448–468.

Fink, C. K. (2005). The predation argument. *Between the Species*, 13(5), 1–16, http://digitalcommons.calpoly.edu/bts/vol13/iss5/3/.

Fink, G. (2016). Stress: Concepts, definition and history. Change History.

Fischer, B. (2018). Individuals in the wild. *Animal Sentience*, 3(23), 170.

Fishcount (2019). Numbers of fish caught in the wild each year. http://fishcount .org.uk/fish-count-estimates-2/numbers-of-fish-caught-from-the-wild-each-year

Fix, A. S., Waterhouse, C., Greiner, E. C., & Stoskopf, M. K. (1988). Plasmodium relictum as a cause of avian malaria in wild-caught Magellanic penguins (*Spheniscus magellanicus*). *Journal of Wildlife Diseases*, 24(4), 610–619.

Fjellström, R. (2002). Specifying speciesism. *Environmental Values*,11(1), 63–74. (2003). Is Singer's ethics speciesist? *Environmental Values*, 12(1), 71–90.

Flatt, T., & Heyland, A. (Eds.). (2011). *Mechanisms of life history evolution: The genetics and physiology of life history traits and trade-offs*. Oxford University Press.

Font, A., Roura, X., Fondevila, D., Closa, J. M., Mascort, J., & Ferrer, L. (1996). Canine mucosal leishmaniasis. *Journal of the American Animal Hospital Association*, 32(2), 131–137.

Fox, H. E., White, S. A., Kao, M. H., & Russell, D. F. (1997). Stress and dominance in a social fish. *Journal of Neuroscience*, 17(16), 6463–6469.

Fox, M. A. (1999). *Deep vegetarianism*. Temple University Press.

Francione, G. L. (1995). *Animals, property, and the law*. Temple University Press. (2000). *Introduction to animal rights: Your child or the dog?* Temple University Press.
(2008). *Animals as persons: Essays on the abolition of animal exploitation*. Columbia University Press.

Francis, L., & Norman, R. (1978). Some animals are more equal than others. *Philosophy*, 53, 507–527.

Franklin, J. H. (2005). *Animal rights and moral philosophy*. Columbia University Press.

Fraser, D. (2008). Understanding animal welfare. *Acta Veterinaria Scandinavica*, 50(1), 1–7.

French, P. A., & Wettstein, H. K. (Eds.). (2000). *Life and death: Metaphysics and ethics*. Blackwell.

Froese, R., & Luna, S. (2004). No relationship between fecundity and annual reproductive rate in bony fish. *Acta Ichthyologica et Piscatoria*, 34, 11–20.

Frey, R. G. (1988). Moral standing, the value of lives, and speciesism. *Between the Species*, 4(3), 10.

Gaard, G. (Ed.). (1993) *Ecofeminism: Women, animals, nature*. Temple University Press.

Galloway, J. A., Green, S. D., Stevens, M., & Kelley, L. A. (2020). Finding a signal hidden among noise: How can predators overcome camouflage strategies? *Philosophical Transactions of the Royal Society B*, 375(1802), 20190478.

Garner. R. (2005). *Animal ethics*. Polity.

Garrabou, J., Coma, R., Bensoussan, N., Bally, M., Chevaldonné, P., Cigliano, M., ... & Cerrano, C. (2009). Mass mortality in Northwestern Mediterranean rocky benthic communities: Effects of the 2003 heat wave. *Global Change Biology*, 15(5), 1090–1103.

Garrido, J. M., Sevilla; I. A., Beltrán-Beck, B., Minguijón, E., Ballesteros, C., Galindo, R. C., ... Gortázar, C. (2011). Protection against tuberculosis in

Eurasian wild boar vaccinated with heat-inactivated *Mycobacterium bovis*. *Public Library of Science One*, *6*, 1–10.

Gheaus, A. (2013). The feasibility constraint on the concept of justice. *The Philosophical Quarterly*, *63*(252), 445–464.

Gilabert, P. (2012). *From global poverty to global equality: A philosophical exploration*. Oxford University Press on Demand.

Gilabert, P., & Lawford-Smith, H. (2012). Political feasibility: A conceptual exploration. *Political Studies*, *60*(4), 809–825.

Gilg, O., Hanski, I., & Sittler, B. (2003). Cyclic dynamics in a simple vertebrate predator-prey community. *Science*, *302*(5646), 866–868.

Gloor, 2019 [2016]. The case for suffering-focused ethics. *Center on Long-Term Risk*. https://longtermrisk.org/the-case-for-suffering-focused-ethics.

Glover, J. (1977). *Causing death and saving lives*. Penguin Books.

Godfrey-Smith, W. (1979). The value of wilderness. *Environmental Ethics*, *1*(4), 309–319.

Godfroid, J., & Käsbohrer, A. (2002). Brucellosis in the European Union and Norway at the turn of the twenty-first century. *Veterinary Microbiology*, *90* (1–4), 135–145.

Godlovitch, R. (1971). Animals and morals. *Philosophy*, *46*(175), 23–33.

Godlovitch, S., Godlovitch, R., & Harris, J. (Eds.). (1971). *Animals, men and morals: An inquiry into the maltreatment of non-humans*. Taplinger.

Gompertz, L. (1997 [1824]) *Moral inquiries on the situation of man and of brutes*. Edwin Mellen Press.

Goodall, J. (1986). *The chimpanzees of Gombe*. Harvard University Press.

Goodpaster, K. E. (1978). On being morally considerable. *Journal of Philosophy*, *75*(6), 308–325.

Gould, S. J. (1994). Nonmoral nature. *Hen's teeth and horse's toes: Further reflections in natural history* (pp. 32–44). W. W. Norton.

Graczyk, T. M., Fayer, R., Trout, J. M., Lewis, E. J., Farley, C. A., Sulaiman, I., & Lal, A. A. (1998). *Giardia* sp. cysts and infectious *Cryptosporidium parvum* oocysts in the feces of migratory Canada geese (*Branta canadensis*). *Applied Environmental Microbiology*, *64*(7), 2736–2738.

Gray, J. (2017). *Zoo ethics: The challenges of compassionate conservation*. Sciro Publishing.

(2018). Challenges of compassionate conservation. *Journal of Applied Animal Welfare Science*, *21*(sup1), 34–42.

Gregory, N. G. (2004). *Physiology and behaviour of animal suffering*. Blackwell.

Griffin, A. S., Callen, A., Klop-Toker, K., Scanlon, R. J., & Hayward, M. W. (2020). Compassionate conservation clashes with conservation biology: Should empathy, compassion, and deontological moral principles drive conservation practice? *Frontiers in Psychology*, *11*, 139.

Griffin, D. R. (1981). *The question of animal awareness: Evolutionary continuity of mental experience*. William Kaufman.

(1992). *Animal minds: Beyond cognition to consciousness*. Chicago University Press.

Griffin, J. (1986). *Well-being: Its meaning, measurement, and moral importance.* Oxford University Press.

Groff, Z., & Ng, Y. K. (2019). Does suffering dominate enjoyment in the animal kingdom? An update to welfare biology. *Biology & Philosophy, 34*(4), 40.

Guinet, C., Domenici, P., de Stephanis, R., Barrett-Lennard, L., Ford, J. K. B., & Verborgh, P. (2007). Killer whale predation on bluefin tuna: Exploring the hypothesis of the endurance-exhaustion technique. *Marine Ecology Progress Series, 347,* 111–119.

Guldemond, R., & Van Aarde, R. (2008). A meta-analysis of the impact of African elephants on savanna vegetation. *The Journal of Wildlife Management, 72*(4), 892–899.

Gulland, F. M. (1999). Stranded seals: Important sentinels. *Journal of the American Veterinary Medical Association, 214*(8), 1191–1192.

Hadley, J. (2006). The duty to aid nonhuman animals in dire need. *Journal of Applied Philosophy, 23*(4), 445–451.

 (2015). *Animal property rights: A theory of habitat rights for wild animals.* Lexington Books.

Hargrove, E. C. (1985). The role of rules in ethical decision making. *Inquiry, 28* (1–4),3–42.

Hargrove, E. C. (Ed.). (1992). *The animal rights/environmental ethics debate: The environmental perspective.* State University of New York Press.

Hartley-Parkinson, R. (2011, November 11st). Saved from a muddy grave: Baby elephant and its mother pulled from lagoon where they got stuck because they wouldn't be separated. *Daily Mail.* www.dailymail.co.uk/news/article-2059502/Baby-elephant-mother-pulled-muddy-grave-conservation-workers-Zambia.html#ixzz3xUL9ea9a.

Haslanger, S. (2000). Gender and race: (What) are they? (What) do we want them to be? *Nous, 34*(1), 31–55.

 (2006). What good are our intuitions? Philosophical analysis and social kinds. *Proceedings of the Aristotelian Society, 80*(1), 89–118.

Hatcher, M. J., Dick, J. T., & Dunn, A. M. (2014). Parasites that change predator or prey behaviour can have keystone effects on community composition. *Biology Letters, 10*(1), 20130879.

Haynes, R. P. (2008). *Animal welfare: Competing conceptions and their ethical implications.* Springer.

Heathwood, C. (2006). Desire satisfactionism and hedonism. *Philosophical Studies, 128*(3), 539–563.

Hecht, L. B. B. (2019). Accounting for demography in the assessment of wild animal welfare. bioRxiv, 819565.

Hennessy, M. B., Deak, T., & Schiml-Webb, P. A. (2001). Stress-induced sickness behaviors: An alternative hypothesis for responses during maternal separation. *Developmental Psychobiology, 39*(2), 76–83.

Henning, J., Schnitzler, F. R., Pfeiffer, D. U., & Davies, P. (2005). Influence of weather conditions on fly abundance and its implications for transmission of rabbit haemorrhagic disease virus in the North Island of New Zealand. *Medical and Veterinary Entomology, 19*(3), 251–262.

Hettinger, N. (1994). Valuing predation in Rolston's environmental ethics: Bambi lovers versus tree huggers. *Environmental Ethics, 16*(1), 3–20.

Hik, D. S. (1995). Does risk of predation influence population dynamics? Evidence from cyclic decline of snowshoe hares. *Wildlife Research, 22*(1), 115–129.

Hillegass, M. A., Waterman, J. M., & Roth, J. D. (2010). Parasite removal increases reproductive success in a social African ground squirrel. *Behavioral Ecology, 21* (4), 696–700.

Hirschman, A. O. (1991). *The rhetoric of reaction*, Harvard University Press.

Holtug, N. (2007). Equality for animals. In Ryberg, J., Petersen, T. S., & Wolf, C. (Eds.) *New waves in applied ethics* (p. 1–24). Palgrave Macmillan.

Hom, C., & May, R. (2013). Moral and semantic innocence. *Analytic Philosophy, 54*(3), 293–313.

(2018). Pejoratives as fiction. In Sosa, D. (Ed.) *Bad words* (pp. 108–131). Oxford University Press.

Horta, O. (2010a). Debunking the idyllic view of natural processes: Population dynamics and suffering in the wild, *Télos, 17*(1), 73–88.

(2010b). What is speciesism? *Journal of Agricultural and Environmental Ethics, 23*(3), 243–266.

(2010c). Interés en vivir y complejidad psicológica: un criterio transespecífico. *La Laguna: Revista de Filosofía, 26*, 109–122.

(2010d). The ethics of the ecology of fear against the nonspeciesist paradigm: A shift in the aims of intervention in nature. *Between the Species, 13*(10), 163–187. http://digitalcommons.calpoly.edu/bts/vol13/iss10/10/.

(2013). Zoopolis, intervention and the state of nature. *Law, Ethics and Philosophy, 1*, 113–125.

(2014). The scope of the argument from species overlap. *Journal of Applied Philosophy, 31*(2), 142–154.

(2014). Egalitarianism and animals. *Between the Species, 19*(1), 5.

(2017a). Animal suffering in nature: The case for intervention. *Environmental Ethics, 39*(3), 261–279.

(2017b). Why the concept of moral status should be abandoned. *Ethical Theory and Moral Practice, 20*(4), 899–910.

(2018). Moral considerability and the argument from relevance. *Journal of Agricultural and Environmental Ethics, 31*(3), 369–388.

Horta, O., & Albersmeier, F. (2020). Defining speciesism. *Philosophy Compass, 15* (11), 1–9.

Howe, F. P. (1992). Effects of *Protocalliphora braueri* (Diptera: Calliphoridae): Parasitism and inclement weather on nestling sage thrashers. *Journal of Wildife Diseases, 28*(1), 141.

Hu, C., Rio, R. V., Medlock, J., Haines, L. R., Nayduch, D., Savage, A. F., . . . & Aksoy, S. (2008). Infections with immunogenic trypanosomes reduce tsetse reproductive fitness: Potential impact of different parasite strains on vector population structure. *PLoS Neglected Tropical Diseases, 2*(3), e192.

Hu, X., Margolis, H. S., Purcell, R. H., Ebert, J., & Robertson, B. H. (2000). Identification of hepatitis B virus indigenous to chimpanzees. *Proceedings of the National Academy of Sciences, 97*(4), 1661–1664.

Hudson, P. J., Dobson, A. P., & Newborn, D. (1992). Do parasites make prey vulnerable to predation? Red grouse and parasites. *Journal of Animal Ecology, 61*(3), 681–692.

Huntingford, F. A., Adams, C., Braithwaite, V. A., Kadri, S., Pottinger, T. G., Sandøe, P., & Turnbull, J. F. (2006). Current issues in fish welfare. *Journal of Fish Biology, 68*(2), 332–372.

Hurka, T. (1993) *Perfectionism.* Oxford University Press.

Hursthouse, R. (2011). Virtue ethics and the treatment of animals. *The Oxford Handbook of Animal Ethics,* 119–143.

Hywel-Jones, N. L. (1996). Cordyceps myrmecophila-like fungi infecting ants in the leaf litter of tropical forest in Thailand. *Mycological Research, 100*(5), 613–619.

Indiana Wildlife Disease News (2009). Starvation and malnutrition in wildlife, *Indiana Wildlife Disease News, 4* (1), 1–3.

Ives, A. R., & Murray, D. L. (1997). Can sublethal parasitism destabilize predator-prey population dynamics? A model of snowshoe hares, predators, and parasites. *Journal of Animal Ecology, 66*(2), 265–278.

Jameson, J., Fauci, A.S., Kasper, D.L., Hauser, S.L., Longo, D.L., & Loscalzo, J. (2018). Protozoal and helminthic infections: General considerations. *Harrison's Principles of Internal Medicine, 20e.* McGraw Hill.

Jamieson, D. (1990). Rights, justice and duties to provide assistance: A critique of Regan's theory of rights. *Ethics, 100*(2), 349–362.

(1998). Animal liberation is an environmental ethic. *Environmental Values, 7* (1), 41–57.

(2002). *Morality's progress: Essays on humans, other animals, and the rest of nature.* Oxford University Press.

(Ed.). (1999). *Singer and his critics.* Blackwell.

Jaquet, F. (2019). Is speciesism wrong by definition?. *Journal of Agricultural and Environmental Ethics, 32*(3), 447–458.

(2020). What's wrong with speciesism. *The Journal of Value Inquiry,* 1–14. https://doi.org/10.1007/s10790-020-09781-y

Jasienska, G. (2020). Costs of reproduction and ageing in the human female. *Philosophical Transactions of the Royal Society B, 375*(1811), 20190615.

Jasienska, G., Bribiescas, R. G., Furberg, A. S., Helle, S., & Núñez-de la Mora, A. (2017). Human reproduction and health: An evolutionary perspective. *The Lancet, 390*(10093), 510–520.

Jefferson, T. A., Stacey, P. J., & Baird, R. W. (1991). A review of killer whale interactions with other marine mammals: Predation to co-existence. *Mammal Review, 21*(4), 151–180.

Jensen, M. (2009). The limits of practical possibility. *The Journal of Political Philosophy*, *17*(2), 168–184.

Johannsen, K. (2017). Animal rights and the problem of r-strategists. *Ethical Theory and Moral Practice*, *20*(2), 333–345.

(2020). *Wild animal ethics: The moral and political problem of wild animal suffering*. Routledge.

Johnson, E. (1981). Animal liberation against the land ethic. *Environmental Ethics*, *3*(3), 265–273.

Jones, C. G., Lawton, J. H., & Shachak, M. (1994). Organisms as ecosystem engineers. In *Ecosystem management* (pp. 130–147). Springer.

jones, P. [sic] (2014). Eros and the mechanisms of eco-defense. In Adams, C. J., & Gruen, L. (Eds.) *Ecofeminism: Feminist intersections with other animals and the Earth* (pp. 91–108). Bloomsbury.

Kaszak, I., Planellas, M., & Dworecka-Kaszak, B. (2015). Canine leishmaniosis – an emerging disease. *Annals of Parasitology*, *61*(2), 69–76.

Kagan, S. (2016). What's wrong with speciesism? (Society for Applied Philosophy Annual Lecture 2015). *Journal of Applied Philosophy*, *33*(1), 1–21.

(2019). *How to count animals, more or less*. Oxford University Press.

Kamm, F. M. (1993). *Morality, mortality. Vol I: Death and whom to save from it*. Oxford University Press.

Katz, E. (1996). The problem of ecological restoration. *Environmental Ethics*, *18*(2), 222–224.

Kaufman, F. (1998). Speciesism and the argument from misfortune. *Journal of Applied Philosophy*, *15*(2), 155–163.

Kavaliers, M., & Colwell, D. D. (1995). Reduced spatial learning in mice infected with the nematode, *Heligmosomoides polygyrus*. *Parasitology*, *110*(5), 591–597.

Keeling, P. M. (2008). Does the idea of wilderness need a defence? *Environmental Values*, *17*(4), 505–519.

Kelly, E., Travouillon, K. J., Keleher, J., Gibson-Kueh, S., & Morgan, D. L. (2016). Mammal predation by an ariid catfish in a dryland river of Western Australia. *Journal of Arid Environments*, *135*, 9–11.

Kirkwood, J. K., & Sainsbury, A. W. (1996). Ethics of interventions for the welfare of free-living wild animals. *Animal Welfare*, *5*, 235–243.

Kitaysky, A. S., Piatt, J. F., Wingfield, J. C., & Romano, M. (1999). The adrenocortical stress-response of black-legged kittiwake chicks in relation to dietary restrictions. *Journal of Comparative Physiology B: Biochemical, Systemic, and Environmental Physiology*, *169*(4), 303–310.

Kohl, M. T., Stahler, D. R., Metz, M. C., Forester, J. D., Kauffman, M. J., Varley, N., ... MacNulty, D. R. (2018). Diel predator activity drives a dynamic landscape of fear. *Ecological Monographs*, *88*(4), 638–652.

Koivula, M., Koskela, E., Mappes, T., & Oksanen, T. A. (2003). Cost of reproduction in the wild: Manipulation of reproductive effort in the bank vole. *Ecology*, *84*(2), 398–405.

Koolhas, J. M., De Boer, S. F., De Rutter, A. J., Meerlo, P., & Sgoifo, A. (1997). Social stress in rats and mice. *Acta Physiologica Scandinavica. Supplementum,* *640,* 69–72.

Koolhas, J. M., De Boer, S. F., Meerlo P., Strubbe, J. H., & Bohus, B. (1997). The temporal dynamics of the stress response. *Neuroscience and Biobehavioral Reviews, 21*(6), 775–782.

Korpimäki, E., Brown, P. R., Jacob, J., & Pech, R. P. (2004). The puzzles of population cycles and outbreaks of small mammals solved? *BioScience, 54* (12), 1071–1079.

Korsgaard, C. (2005) Fellow creatures: Kantian ethics and our duties to animals, *The Tanner Lectures on Human Values, 25–26,* 77–110.

Korsgaard, C. M. (2018). *Fellow creatures: Our obligations to the other animals.* Oxford University Press.

Kowalski, K., & Rychlik, L. (2018). The role of venom in the hunting and hoarding of prey differing in body size by the Eurasian water shrew, Neomys fodiens. *Journal of Mammalogy, 99*(2), 351–362.

Kyriazakis, I., & Tolkamp, B. J. (2011). Hunger and thirst. In Appleby, M. C., Mench, J. A., Olsson, I. A. S., & Hughes, B. O. (Eds.), *Animal welfare* (pp. 44–63). CABI.

LaFollette, H., & Shanks, N. (1996). The origin of speciesism. *Philosophy, 71* (275), 41–61.

Lascalles, B. D. X. (1996). Advances in control of pain in animals. *The Veterinary Annual, 36,* 1–15.

Laundré, J. W., Hernández, L., and Altendorf, K. B. (2001). Wolves, elk, and bison: Reestablishing the 'landscape of fear' in Yellowstone National Park, U.S.A. *Canadian Journal of Zoology, 79* (8), 1401–1409.

Laws, R.M. (1970). Elephants as agents of habitat and landscape change in East Africa. *OIKOS, 21,* 1–15.

Leahy, M. (1991). *Against liberation: Putting animals in perspective.* Routledge.

Leggett, H. (2009, August 4). Plague vaccine for prairie dogs could save endangered ferret. *Wired.* www.wired.com/2009/08/prairiedogvax/.

Leopold, A. (1989 [1949]). *A sand county almanac and sketches here and there.* Oxford University Press.

Libersat, F., Delago, A., & Gal, R. (2009). Manipulation of host behavior by parasitic insects and insect parasites. *Annual Review of Entomology, 54,* 189–207.

Lichtenberg, J. (2010). Negative duties, positive duties, and the "new harms". *Ethics, 120*(3), 557–578.

Linkola, P. (2009) *Can life prevail? A radical approach to the environmental crisis.* Integral Tradition Publishing.

Lippert-Rasmussen, K. (2006). The badness of discrimination. *Ethical Theory and Moral Practice, 9*(2), 167–185.

(2014). *Born free and equal? A philosophical inquiry into the nature of discrimination.* Oxford University Press.

Loftin, R. W. (1985). The medical treatment of wild animals. *Environmental Ethics*, *7*(3), 231–239.

Loh, R., Bergfeld, J., Hayes, D., O'Hara, A., Pyecroft, S., Raidal, S., & Sharpe, R. (2006). The pathology of Devil Facial Tumor Disease (DFTD) in Tasmanian Devils (*Sarcophilus harrisii*). *Veterinary Pathology*, *43*(6), 890–895.

Low, P., Panksepp, J., Reiss, D., Edelman, D., Van Swinderen, B., & Koch, C. (2012). *The Cambridge declaration on consciousness*. Cambridge.

Lu, C., Sopory, A., & Whittaker, K. (2010 [2000]). Rana catesbeiana. *Amphibia Web*. https://amphibiaweb.org/cgi/amphib_query?rel-common_name=like&where-scientific_name=rana+catesbeiana&account=amphibiaweb

Ludwig, D. (1945). The effects of atmospheric humidity on animal life. *Physiological Zoology*, *18*(2), 103–135.

Luper, S. (2009). *The philosophy of death*. Cambridge University Press.

MacArthur, R. H., & Wilson, E. O. (1967). *The theory of island biogeography*. Princeton University Press.

MacAskill, W. (2015). *Doing good better: Effective altruism and a radical new way to make a difference*. Guardian Faber.

MacClellan, J. P. (2013). What the wild things are: A critique on Clare Palmer's 'What (if anything) do we owe wild animals? *Between the Species*, 16(1), 53–67. http://digitalcommons.calpoly.edu/bts/vol16/iss1/6/.

Macdonald, J. W., Goater, R., Atkinson, N. K., & Small, J. (1990). Further causes of death in Scottish swans (*Cygnus* spp.). *State Veterinary Journal*, *44* (124), 81–93.

MacInnes, C. D., & LeBer, C. A. (2000). Wildlife management agencies should participate in rabies control. *Wildlife Society Bulletin*, *28*, 1156–1167.

Madhavan Nair, R. (2004, Mach 26). Hunger and thirst haunt wildlife. *The Hindu: Online edition of India's National Newspaper*. www.hindu.com/2004/03/26/stories/2004032608110500.htm.

Malli, H., Kuhn-Nentwig, L., Imboden, H., & Nentwig, W. (1999). Effects of size, motility and paralysation time of prey on the quantity of venom injected by the hunting spider *Cupiennius salei*. *Journal of Experimental Biology*, *202*(15), 2083–2089.

Mannino, A. (2015). Humanitarian intervention in nature: Crucial questions and probable answers. *Relations: Beyond Anthropocentrism*, *3*(1), 109–120.

Marietta, D. E. (1993). Pluralism in environmental ethics. *Topoi*, *12*(1): 69–80.

Marion, P. L., Knight, S. S., Ho, B. K., Guo, Y., Robinson, W. S., & Popper, H. (1984). Liver disease associated with duck hepatitis B virus infection of domestic ducks. *Proceedings of the National Academy of Sciences*, *81*(3), 898–902.

Matheny, G. (2006). Utilitarianism and animals. In: Singer, P. (Ed.), *In defense of animals: The second wave* (pp. 13–25). Blackwell Pub.

Mather, J. A. (2001). Animal suffering: An invertebrate perspective. *Journal of Applied Animal Welfare Science*, *4*(2), 151–156.

McAuliffe, J. R. (1978). *Biological survey and management of sport-hunted bullfrog populations in Nebraska*. Nebraska Game & Parks Commission.

McCallum, H., Tompkins, D. M., Jones, M., Lachish, S., Marvanek, S., Lazenby, B., ... & Hawkins, C. (2007). Distribution and impacts of Tasmanian Devil Facial Tumor Disease. *EcoHealth*, *4*(3), 318–325.

McCauley, S., Rowe, J. L., & Fortin, M.-J. (2011). The deadly effects of 'nonlethal' predators. *Ecology*, *92*(11), 2043–2048.

McCloskey, H. J. (1979). Moral rights and animals. *Inquiry*, 22(1–4), 23–54.

McKinney, F., & Evarts, S. (1998). Sexual coercion in waterfowl and other birds. *Ornithological Monographs*, *49*, 163–195.

McMahan, J. (1988). Death and the value of life. *Ethics*, *99*(1), 32–61.

(1996). Cognitive disability, misfortune, and justice. *Philosophy & Public Affairs*, *25*(1), 3–35.

(2002). *The ethics of killing: Problems at the margins of life*. Oxford University Press.

(2005). Our fellow creatures. *The Journal of Ethics*, *9*(3), 353–380.

(2008). Challenges to human equality. *Journal of Ethics*, *12*(1), 81–104.

(2010a, September 19). The meat eaters. *The New York Times*. http://opinionator.blogs.nytimes.com/2010/09/19/the-meat-eaters/.

(2010b, September 28). A Response. *The New York Times*. http://opinionator.blogs.nytimes.com/2010/09/28/predtors-a-response.

(2015). The moral problem of predation. In Chignell, A., Cuneo, T., & Halteman, M. (Eds.), *Philosophy comes to dinner: Arguments on the ethics of eating* (pp. 268–294). Routledge.

(2016). On 'modal personism'. *Journal of Applied Philosophy*, *33*(1), 26–30.

McNamara, J. M., & Houston, A. I. (1987). Starvation and predation as factors limiting population size. *Ecology*, *68*(5), 1515–1519.

McNulty, S. (2010). Florida sea turtle cold stunning. Wildlife Data Integration Network. Madison, Wisconsin, USA.

McPherson, T. (2014). A case for ethical veganism. *Journal of Moral Philosophy*, *11*(6), 677–703.

Melden, A. I. (1980). *Rights and persons*. University of California Press.

Michigan Department of Natural Resources (2019). Malnutrition and starvation. www.michigan.gov/dnr/0,4570,7-350-79136_79608_85016-26946-,00.html

Milburn, J. (2015). Rabbits, stoats and the predator problem: Why a strong animal rights position need not call for human intervention to protect prey from predators. *Res Publica*, *21*(3), 273–289.

(2017). Nonhuman animals as property holders: An exploration of the Lockean labour-mixing account. *Environmental Values*, *26*(5), 629–648.

Mill, J. S. (1969 [1874]) *Nature*. In *Collected works*, vol. X (pp. 373–402). Routledge and Kegan Paul.

Mill, S. (1902 [1874]). *On nature*. In *Nature, The Utility of Religion and Theism*. The Rationalist Press.

Miller, H. B., & Williams, W. H. (Eds.). (1983). *Ethics and animals*. Humana Press.

Miller, M. W., Swanson, H. M., Wolfe, L. L., Quartarone, F. G., Huwer S. L., Southwick, C. H., & Lukacs, P. M. (2008). Lions and prions and deer demise. *Public Library of Science One*, 3, e4019.

Moberg, G. P., & Mench, J. A. (2000). *The biology of animal stress: Basic principles and implications for animal welfare*. CABI.

Monsó, S. (2019). How to tell if animals can understand death. *Erkenntnis*, 1–20.
(2021). Is predation necessarily amoral? In *Crisis and critique: Philosophical analysis and current events* (pp. 367–382). De Gruyter.

Monsó, S., & Osuna-Mascaró, A. J. (2020). Death is common, so is understanding it: The concept of death in other species. *Synthese*, 1–25.

Mood, A. and Brooke, P. (2012). Estimating the number of farmed fish killed in global aquaculture each year. http://fishcount.org.uk/published/std/fish countstudy2.pdf

Mott, C. L. (2010). Environmental constraints to the geographic expansion of plant and animal species. *Nature Education Knowledge*, 3(10), 72.

Muller, M. N., & Wrangham, R. W. (2009). *Sexual coercion in primates and humans: An evolutionary perspective on male aggression against females*. Harvard University Press.

Murray, D. L., Keith, L. B., & Cary, J. R. (1998). Do parasitism and nutritional status interact to affect production in snowshoe hares? *Ecology*, 79(4), 1209–1222.

Nabi, D. G., Tak, S. R., Kangoo, K. A., & Halwai, M. A. (2009). Increasing incidence of injuries and fatalities inflicted by wild animals in Kashmir. *Injury: International Journal of the Care of the Injured*, 40(1), 87–89.

Naess, A. (1991). Should we try to relieve clear cases of suffering in nature?. *Pan Ecology*, 6(1), 1–5.

Nagel, T. (1970). Death. *Noûs*, 4, 73–80.
(1991). *Equality and partiality*. Oxford University Press.

Narveson, J. (1977). Animal rights. *Canadian Journal of Philosophy*, 7(1), 161–178.

Nelson, L. (1956) *System of ethics*. Yale University Press.

Nelson, M. P. (2010). Teaching holism in environmental ethics. *Environmental Ethics*, 32(1), 33–49.

Nelson, M. P., & Callicott, J. B. (Eds.). (2008). *The wilderness debate rages on: Continuing the great new wilderness debate*. University of Georgia Press.

Nelson, Michael P. (Eds.) (2007). The great new wilderness debate: An overview. In Pojman, L. P., & Pojman, P. (Eds.), *Environmental ethics: Readings in theory and application* (pp. 200–208). Wadsworth.

Ng, Y. K. (2016). How welfare biology and commonsense may help to reduce animal suffering. *Animal Sentience*, 1(7), 1.

Ng, Y.-K. (1995). Towards welfare biology: Evolutionary economics of animal consciousness and suffering. *Biology and Philosophy*, 10, 255–285.

Nobis, N. (2002). Vegetarianism and virtue: Does consequentialism demand *too little? Social Theory and Practice, 28*(1), 135–156.

(2004). Carl Cohen's 'kind' argument for animal rights and against human rights. *Journal of Applied Philosophy, 21*(1), 43–59.

Norcross, A. (2004). Puppies, pigs, and people: Eating meat and marginal cases. *Philosophical Perspectives, 18*, 229–245.

Nozick, R. (1974). *Anarchy, state and utopia*. Basil Backwell.

Nussbaum, M. C. (2004). Beyond compassion and humanity: Justice for nonhuman animals. In Sustein, C., & Nussbaum, M. C. (Eds.), *Animal rights: Current debates and new directions* (pp. 299–320). Oxford University Press.

(2006). *Frontiers of justice: Disability, nationality, species membership*. Harvard University Press.

O'Brien, G. D. (2021). Directed Panspermia, wild animal suffering, and the ethics of world-creation. *Journal of Applied Philosophy*. https://doi.org/10.1111/japp.12538

O'Neill, J., Holland, A., & Light, A. (2008). *Environmental values*. Routledge.

O'Neill, O. (1997). Environmental values, anthropocentrism and speciesism. *Environmental Values, 6*, 127–142.

Ottenweller, J. E. (2000). Animals models (nonprimate) for human stress. *Encyclopedia of Stress, 1*, 200–205.

Packer, C., Ikanda, D., Kissui, B., & Kushnir, H. (2005). Conservation biology: Lion attacks on humans in Tanzania. *Nature, 436*(7053), 927–928.

Paez, E. (2017). Interests without desire, badness without interests: The disvalue of death in Singer's hedonistic utilitarianism. In Dardenne, E., Giroux, V., & Utria, E. (Eds.), *Libération Animale, 40 ans plus tard (Animal Liberation, 40 years on)*. Rennes University Press.

(2021). A republic for all sentients: Social freedom without free will. *Pacific Philosophical Quarterly*. https://doi.org/10.1111/papq.12351

Palmer, C. A. (2010). *Animal ethics in context*. Columbia University Press.

(2013). What (if anything) do we owe wild animals? *Between the Species, 16*, 15–38, http://digitalcommons.calpoly.edu/bts/vol16/iss1/4/.

(2015). Against the view that we are usually required to assist wild animals, *Relations: Beyond Anthropocentrism, 3*(1), 203–210.

Parfit, D. (1995). *Equality or priority*. University of Kansas.

Parfit. D. (1984). *Reasons and persons*. Oxford University Press.

(2004 [1986]). Overpopulation and the quality of life. In Ryberg, J., & Tännsjö, T. (Eds.), *The repugnant conclusion: Essays on population ethics* (pp. 7–22). Kluwer.

Parmesan, C., Root, T. L., & Willig, M. R. (2000). Impacts of extreme weather and climate on terrestrial biota. *Bulletin of the American Meteorological Society, 81*(3), 443–450.

Paterson, D., & Ryder, R. D. (Eds.) (1979). *Animal rights – A symposium*. Centaur Press.

Pearce, D. (2015 [2009]). Reprogramming predators. The Hedonistic Imperative. www.hedweb.com/abolitionist-project/reprogramming-predators.html

(2015). A welfare state for elephants? A case study of compassionate steward-ship. *Relations: Beyond Anthropocentrism, 3*(2), 133–152.

Pedersen, A. B., Jones, K. E., Nunn, C. I., & Altizer, S. (2007). Infectious diseases and extinction risk in wild mammals. *Conservation Biology, 21*(5), 1269–1279.

Pembury Smith, M. Q., & Ruxton, G. D. (2020). Camouflage in predators. *Biological Reviews, 95*(5), 1325–1340.

Pepper, A. (2020). Glass panels and peepholes: Nonhuman animals and the right to privacy. *Pacific Philosophical Quarterly, 101*(4), 628–650.

Persson, I. (1993). A basis for (interspecies) equality. In Cavalieri, P., & Singer, P. (Eds.), *The Great Ape Project: Equality beyond humanity* (pp. 183–193). St. Martin's Press.

Petrinovich, L. (1999). *Darwinian Dominion: Animal welfare and human interests.* MIT Press.

Pianka, E. R. (1970). On r- and K-selection. *The American Naturalist, 104*(940), 592–597.

Pitman, R. L., Totterdell, J. A., Fearnbach, H., Ballance, L. T., Durban, J. W., & Kemps, H. (2015). Whale killers: Prevalence and ecological implications of killer whale predation on humpback whale calves off Western Australia. *Marine Mammal Science, 31*(2), 629–657.

Pluhar, E. B. (1995). *Beyond prejudice: The moral significance of human and nonhuman animals.* Duke University Press.

Plumwood, V. (1995). Human vulnerability and the experience of being prey. *Quadrant, 39*(3), 29–34.

Poliza, M. (2002). Elephant calf being eaten alive. *Flickr.* www.flickr.com/photos/poliza/183530778/.

Poole, J. (1998). An exploration of a commonality between ourselves and ele-phants. *Etica & Animali, 9*(98), 85–110.

Pounds, J. A., Bustamante, M. R., Coloma, L. A., Consuegra, J. A., Fogden, M. P. L., Foster, P. N., ... Young, B. E. (2006). Widespread amphibian extinctions from epidemic disease driven by global warming. *Nature, 439* (7073), 161–167.

Prevedello, J. A., Dickman, C. R., Vieira, M. V., & Vieira, E. M. (2013). Population responses of small mammals to food supply and predators: A global meta-analysis. *Journal of Animal Ecology, 82*(5), 927–936.

Price, E. O. (1999). Behavioral development in animals undergoing domestica-tion. *Applied Animal Behaviour Science, 65*(3), 254–271.

Proaktor, G., Coulson, T., & Milner-Gulland, E. J. (2008). The demographic consequences of the cost of reproduction in ungulates. *Ecology, 89*(9), 2604–2611.

Prugnolle, F., Durand, P., Neel, C., Ollomo, B., Ayala, F. J., Arnathau, C., ... & Renaud, F. (2010). African great apes are natural hosts of multiple related malaria species, including Plasmodium falciparum. *Proceedings of the National Academy of Sciences, 107*(4), 1458–1463.

Prugnolle, F., Rougeron, V., Becquart, P., Berry, A., Makanga, B., Rahola, N., ... Renaud, F. (2013). Diversity, host switching and evolution of Plasmodium vivax infecting African great apes. *Proceedings of the National Academy of Sciences, 110*(20), 8123–8128.

Pryce, C. R., Rüedi-Bettschen, D., Dettling, A. C., & Feldon, J. (2002). Early life stress: Long-term physiological impact in rodents and primates. *News in Physiological Sciences: An International Journal of Physiology Produced Jointly by the International Union of Physiological Sciences and the American Physiological Society, 17*(4), 150–155.

Pyecroft, S. B., Pearse, A.-M., Loh, R., Swift, K., Belov, K., Fox, N., ... Moore, R. J. (2007). Towards a case definition for Devil Facial Tumour Disease: What is it? *EcoHealth, 4*(3), 346–351.

Rachels, J. (1990). *Created from animals: The moral implications of darwinism.* Oxford University Press.

Ramp, D., & Bekoff, M. (2015). Compassion as a practical and evolved ethic for conservation. *BioScience, 65*(3), 323–327.

Raterman, T. (2008). An environmentalist's lament on predation. *Environmental Ethics, 30*(4), 417–434.

Rawls, J. (1999). *A theory of justice: Revised edition.* Harvard University Press.

Raz, J. (1986) *The morality of freedom.* Oxford University Press.

Regan, T. (1975). The moral basis of vegetarianism. *Canadian Journal of Philosophy, 5*(2), 181–214.

(1983). Animal rights, human wrongs. In *Ethics and animals* (pp. 19–43). Humana Press.

(2004 [1983]). *The case for animal rights.* University of California Press.

Republic of Namibia (2004). Transfer of the Namibian Population of Nile Crocodile (Crocodylus niloticus) to Appendix II. CITES COP13 Proposal 25, Geneva.

Rethink Priorities (2020). Research summary: The intensity of valenced experiences. https://rethinkpriorities.org/publications/research-summary-the-intensity-of-valenced-experience-across-species

Reznick, D., Bryant M. J., & Bashey, F. (2002). *r*-and *K*-selection revisited: The role of population regulation in life-history evolution. *Ecology, 83*(6), 1509–1520.

Robinson Jr., E. J. (1947). Notes on the Life History of *Leucochloridium fuscostriatum* n. sp. provis. (Trematoda: Brachylaemidae). *Journal of Parasitology, 33*(6), 467–475.

Roff, D. A. (1992). *Evolution of life histories: Theory and analysis.* Springer.

Rollin, B. E. (1981). *Animal rights and human morality.* Prometheus Books.

(1989). *The unheeded cry: Animal consciousness, animal pain and science.* Oxford University Press.

Rolston III, H. (1992). Disvalues in nature. *The Monist, 75*(2), 250–278.

(1999). Respect for life: Counting what Singer finds of no account. In Jamieson, D. (Ed.), *Singer and his critics* (pp. 247–268). Blackwell.

Romero, L. M., Reed, J. M., & Wingfield, J. C. (2000). Effects of weather on corticosterone responses in wild free-living passerine birds. *General and Comparative Endocrinology, 118*(1), 113–122.

Roser, M., Ritchie, H., & Ortiz-Ospina, E. (2013). World Population Growth. Published online at OurWorldInData.org. Retrieved from: https://ourworldindata.org/world-population-growth'.

Rossow, L. M. (1981). Why do species matter? *Environmental Ethics, 3*(2), 101–112.

Rothgerber, H. (2020). Meat-related cognitive dissonance: A conceptual framework for understanding how meat eaters reduce negative arousal from eating animals. *Appetite, 146*, 104511.

Rowlands, M. (1998) *Animal rights: A philosophical defence.* MacMillan Press.
(2002) *Animals like us.* Verso.

Russell, B. (1977). On the relative strictness of negative and positive duties. *American Philosophical Quarterly, 14*(2), 87–97.

Ryder, R. D. (1975) *Victims of science: The use of animals in research.* Davis-Poynter.

Ryder, R. (1983). *Victims of science* (revised edition). Fontwell, National Anti-Vivisection Society.
(2010 [1970]). Speciesism: The original leaflet. *Critical Society, 2,* 1–2.

Sæther, B. E., Coulson, T., Grøtan, V., Engen, S., Altwegg, R., Armitage, K. B., ... Festa-Bianchet, M. (2013). How life history influences population dynamics in fluctuating environments. *The American Naturalist, 182*(6), 743–759

Sagoff, M. (1984). Animal liberation and environmental ethics: Bad marriage, quick divorce. *Osgoode Hall Law Journal, 22,* 297–307.

Salt, H. S. (1980 [1892]). *Animals' rights: Considered in relation to social progress.* Open Gate Press.

Salzman, A. G. (1982). The selective importance of heat stress in gull nest location. *Ecology, 63*(3), 742–751.

Sandøe, P., & Simonsen, H. B. (1992). Assessing animal welfare: Where does science end and philosophy begin? *Animal Welfare, 1*(4), 257–267.

Sapolsky, R. M. (1986). Endocrine and behavioral correlates of drought in wild olive baboons (*Papio anubis*). *American Journal of Primatology, 11*(3), 217–227.
(2004). Social status and health in humans and other animals. *Annual Review of Anthropology, 33,* 393–418.
(2005). The influence of social hierarchy on primate health. *Science, 308*(5722), 648–652.

Sapolszky, R. (1990). Stress in the wild. *Scientific American, 262*(1), 116–123.

Sapontzis, S. F. (1982). The moral significance of interests. *Environmental Ethics, 4*(4), 345–358.
(1984). Predation. *Ethics and Animals, 5*(2), 27–38.
(1987). *Morals, reason, and animals.* Temple University Press.

(1993). Aping persons – pro and con. In Cavalieri, P., & Singer, P. (Eds.), *The Great Ape Project: Equality beyond humanity* (pp. 269–277). St. Martin's Press.

Sapontzis, S. F. (Ed.). (2004). *Food for thought: The debate over eating meat.* Prometheus.

Scarre, G. (2007). *Death.* Acumen.

Schmidt, M. (1986 [1985]). Elephants (Proboscidae). In Fowler, M. E. (Ed.), *Zoo & wild animal medicine* (pp. 883–923). WB Saunders & Co.

Schmidtz, D. (1998). Are all species equal? *Journal of Applied Philosophy, 15*(1), 57–67.

Schweitzer, A. (1973 [1923]). *Culture and ethics.* Progress Publishers.

Scruton, R. (1996). *Animal rights and wrongs.* Metro.

Segelson, C. (2010). *Record cold leads to record numbers of manatee deaths.* Florida Fish and Wildlife Conservation Commission.

Seppälä, O., Karvonen, A., & Valtonen, E. T. (2004). Parasite-induced change in host behaviour and susceptibility to predation in an eye fluke-fish interaction. *Animal Behaviour, 68*(2), 257–263.

Shannon, G., Druce, D.J., Page, B.R., Eckhardt, H.C., Grant, R., & Slotow, R. (2008). The utilization of large savanna trees by elephant in southern Kruger National Park. *Journal of Tropical Ecology, 24*(3), 281–289.

Shelton, J.-A. (2004). Killing animals that don't fit in: Moral dimensions of habitat restoration. *Between the Species, 13*(4), 1–21 http://digitalcommons .calpoly.edu/bts/vol13/iss4/3/.

Shiverly, C. A.; Laber-Laird, K., & Anton, R. F. (1997). Behavior and physiology of social stress and depression in female cynomolgus monkeys. *Biological Psychiatry, 41*(8), 871–882.

Sibly, R. M., & Hone, J. (2002). Population growth rate and its determinants: An overview. *Philosophical Transactions of the Royal Society of London. Series B: Biological Sciences, 357*(1425), 1153–1170.

Sideleau, B. (2016). Summary of worldwide crocodilian attacks for 2015. In *Proceedings of 23rd Working Meeting of the Crocodile Specialist Group of the Species Survival Commission of IUCN2014 May* (pp. 26–30).

Sidgwick, H. (1996 [1874]). *The methods of ethics.* Thoemmes Press.

Silverstein, H. S. (1980). The evil of death. *Journal of Philosophy, 77*(7), 401–424.

Simmons, A. (2009). Animals, predators, the right to life and the duty to save lives. *Ethics & the Environment, 14,* 15–27.

Simpson, V. R. (2002). Wild animals as reservoirs of infectious diseases in the UK. *The Veterinary Journal, 163*(2), 128–146.

Sinclair, A., & Krebs, C. J. (2002). Complex numerical responses to top–down and bottom–up processes in vertebrate populations. *Philosophical Transactions of the Royal Society of London, 357*(1425), 1221–1231.

Sinclair, A. R. E., & Arcese, P. (1995). Population consequences of predation-sensitive foraging: The Serengeti wildebeest. *Ecology, 76*(3), 882–891.

Singer. P. (1971) Famine, affluence, and morality. *Philosophy and Public Affairs, 1,* 229–243.

Singer, P. (1975). *Animal liberation: Towards an end to man's inhumanity to animals*. Granada Publishing Ltd.

(1997). The drowning child and the expanding circle. *New Internationalist, 289*, http://newint.org/features/1997/04/05/drowning/

(2002). A response to Martha Nussbaum. *Utilitarian.net*, www.utilitarian.net/singer/by/20021113.htm.

(2009 [1974]). *Animal liberation*. HarperCollins.

(2011 [1979]). *Practical ethics*. Cambridge University Press.

(2016). Afterword. In Visak, T., & Garner, R. (Eds.), *The ethics of killing animals* (pp. 229–235). Oxford University Press.

(2016). Why speciesism is wrong: A response to K. Agan. *Journal of Applied Philosophy, 33*(1), 31–35.

Slate, D., Rupprecht, C. E., Rooney, J. A., Donovan, D., Lein, D. H., & Chipman, R. B. (2005). Status of oral rabies vaccination in wild carnivores in the United States. *Virus Research, 111*(1), 68–76.

Smith, A. (1970). Frostbite, hypothermia, and resuscitation after freezing. In Smith, A. (Ed.), *Current trends in cryobiology* (pp. 181–208). Springer.

Smith, B. L. (2001). Winter feeding of elk in western North America. *Journal of Wildlife Management, 65*, 173–190.

Smith, J. A. (1991). A question of pain in invertebrates. *Institute for Laboratory Animal Research Journal, 33*(1–2), 25–32.

Smuts, B. B., & Smuts, R. W. (1993). Male aggression and sexual coercion of females in nonhuman primates and other mammals: Evidence and theoretical implications. *Advances in the Study of Behavior, 22*(22), 1–63.

Soryl, A. A., Moore, A. J., Seddon, P. J., & King, M. R. (2021). The case for welfare biology. *Journal of Agricultural and Environmental Ethics, 34*(2), 1–25.

Sotala, K., & Gloor, L. (2017). Superintelligence as a cause or cure for risks of astronomical suffering. *Informatica, 41*(4), 389–400.

Soulsby, E. J. L. (1982). Helminths, arthropods and protozoa of domesticated animals. (Ed. 7), xi + 809 pp. 44. Baillière Tindall, London, United Kingdom.

Spiegel, M. (1988). *The dreaded comparison: Human and animal slavery*. Heretic Books.

Stearns, S. C. (1992). *The evolution of life histories*. Oxford University Press.

Steiner, G. (2005). *Anthropocentrism and its discontents: The moral status of animals in the history of western philosophy*. University of Pittsburgh Press.

Sterba, J. P. (2011). Biocentrism defended. *Ethics, Policy & Environment, 14*(2), 167–169.

Stevens, M. (2007). Predator perception and the interrelation between different forms of protective coloration. *Proceedings of the Royal Society B: Biological Sciences, 274*(1617), 1457–1464.

Stone, Christopher D. (1987). *Earth and other ethics: The case for moral pluralism*. Harper and Row.

Stzutenbaker, C. D., Brown, K., & Lobpries, D. (1986). Special report: An assessment of the accuracy of documenting waterfowl die offs in a Texas coastal marsh. In Feierabend, J. S., & Russell, A. B. (Eds.), *Lead poisoning in wild waterfowl, a workshop* (pp. 88–95). National Wildlife Federation.

Suits, D. B. (2001). Why death is not bad for the one who died. *American Philosophical Quarterly, 38*(1), 69–84.

Sumner, L. W. (1996). *Welfare, happiness, and ethics.* Oxford University Press.

Sures, B., Nachev, M., Pahl, M., Grabner, D., & Selbach, C. (2017). Parasites as drivers of key processes in aquatic ecosystems: Facts and future directions. *Experimental Parasitology, 180,* 141–147.

Sustein, C., & Nussbaum, M. C. (Eds.). (2004). *Animal rights: Current debates and new directions.* Oxford University Press.

Sweitzer, R. A. (1996). Predation or starvation: Consequences of foraging decisions by porcupines (*Erethizon dorsatum*). *Journal of Mammalogy, 77*(4), 1068–1077

Sztybel, D. (2008). Animals as persons. In Castricano, J. (Ed.), *Animal subjects: An ethical reader in a Posthuman World* (pp. 241–257). Wilfrid Laurier University Press.

Takahata, Y., Hasegawa, T., & Nishida, T. (1984). Chimpanzee predation in the Mahale Mountains from August 1979 to May 1982. *International Journal of Primatology, 5*(3), 213–233.

Tanner, J. (2011a) The argument from marginal cases: Is species a relevant difference? *Croatian Journal of Philosophy,* 11, 225–235.

(2011b). Rowlands, Rawlsian justice and animal experimentation. *Ethical Theory and Moral Practice, 14*(5), 569–587.

(2013). Contractarianism and secondary direct moral standing for marginal humans and animals. *Res Publica, 19*(2), 141–156.

Taylor, P. (1981). The ethics of respect for nature. *Environmental Ethics, 3*(3), 197–218.

(1983). In defense of biocentrism. *Environmental Ethics, 5*(3), 237–243.

(1986). *Respect for nature.* Princeton University Press.

Taylor, S. (2017). *Beasts of burden: Animal and disability liberation.* The New Press.

Temkin, L. S. (2012). *Rethinking the good: Moral ideals and the nature of practical reasoning.* Oxford University Press.

Thomas, F, Poulin, R., & Brodeur, J. (2010). Host manipulation by parasites: A multidimensional phenomenon. *Oikos, 119*(8), 1217–1223.

Thomas, C. D., Singer, M. C., & Boughton, D. A. (1996). Catastrophic extinction of population sources in a butterfly metapopulation. *The American Naturalist, 148*(6), 957–975.

Thornhill, R., & Morris, M. (2006). Animal liberationist responses to non-anthropogenic animal suffering. *Worldviews: Global Religions, Culture, and Ecology, 10*(3), 355–379.

Todd, B. (2013). A framework for strategically selecting a cause. *80000hours.org.* https://80000hours.org/2013/12/a-framework-for-strategically-selecting-a-cause/

Tomasik, B. (2015a [2009]). The importance of wild-animal suffering. *Relations: Beyond Anthropocentrism, 3*(1), 133–152.

Tomasik (2015b). Estimating aggregate wild-animal suffering from reproductive age and births per female. *Essays on Reducing Suffering.* http://reducingsufferi ng.org/estimating-aggregate-wild-animal-suffering-from-reproductive-age-and-birthsper-female/#_blank.

Torres, E. (2012, February 16). Should we vaccinate wild apes? *Global Animal.* http://www.globalanimal.org/2012/02/16/should-we-vaccinate-wild-apes/ 66511/.

Torres, M. (2015). The case for intervention in nature on behalf of animals: A critical review of the main arguments against intervention. *Relations: Beyond Anthropocentrism, 3,* 33–49.

Unger, P. (1996). *Living high and letting die: Our illusion of innocence.* Oxford University Press.

Vallentyne, P. (2005). Of mice and men: Equality and animals. *Journal of Ethics, 9*(3–4), 403–433.

Varner, G. (1998). *In nature's interests? Interests, animal rights, and environmental ethics.* Oxford University Press.

  (2012). *Personhood, ethics, and animal cognition: Situating animals in Hare's two level utilitarianism.* Oxford University Press.

  (2017). Biocentric individualism. In Robin Attfield, *The ethics of the environment* (pp. 287–299). Routledge.

Verbitski, A., Dodfel, D., & Zhang, N. (2020). Rodent models of post-traumatic stress disorder: Behavioral assessment. *Translational psychiatry, 10*(1), 1–28.

Verhulst, P.-F. (1838). Notice sur la loi que la population poursuit dans son accroissement. *Correspondance mathématique et physique, 10,* 113–121.

Visak, T. (2013). *Killing happy animals: Explorations in utilitarian ethics.* Palgrave MacMillan.

Visak, T., & Garner, R. (Eds.) (2016). *The ethics of killing animals.* Oxford University Press.

Waldau, P. (2001). *The specter of speciesism: Buddhist and Christian views of animals.* Oxford University Press.

Waldhorn, D. R. (2019). Toward a new framework for understanding human–wild animal relations. *American Behavioral Scientist, 63*(8), 1080–1100.

Wellman, C. H. (1996). Liberalism, samaritanism, and political legitimacy. *Philosophy & Public Affairs, 25*(3), 211–237.

  (2001). Toward a liberal theory of political obligation. *Ethics, 111*(4), 735–759.

Wenz, P. S. (1988). *Environmental justice.* SUNY Press.

White, A. (1989). Why animals cannot have rights. In Regan, T., & Singer, P. (Eds.), *Animal rights and human obligations* (pp. 119–121). Prentice Hall.

White, T. (2007). *In defense of dolphins: The new moral frontier.* Blackwell.

White, T. C. R. (2008). The role of food, weather and climate in limiting the abundance of animals. *Biological Reviews, 83*(3), 227–248.

Wiepkema, P. R., & van Adrichem, P. W. M. (Eds.) (1987). *Biology of stress in farm animals: An integrative approach.* Kluwer.

Wigger, E., Kuhn-Nentwig, L., & Nentwig, W. (2002). The venom optimisation hypothesis: A spider injects large venom quantities only into difficult prey types. *Toxicon, 40*(6), 749–752.

Williams, B. A. O. (1985). *Ethics and the limits of philosophy.* Fontana.

(2006). The human prejudice. In A. W. Moore, *Philosophy as a humanistic discipline* (pp. 135–152). Princeton University Press.

Wilson, S. (2005). The species-norm account of moral status. *Between the Species, 13*(5), 1–29, http://digitalcommons.calpoly.edu/bts/vol13/iss5/7/.

Wizen, G., & Gasith, A. (2011). Predation of amphibians by carabid beetles of the genus Epomis found in the central coastal plain of Israel. *ZooKeys, 100,* 181–191.

Wobeser, G. A. (2013). *Investigation and management of disease in wild animals.* Springer Science & Business Media.

Wolff, J. O., & Sherman, P. W. (Eds.). (2008). *Rodent societies: An ecological and evolutionary perspective.* University of Chicago Press.

World Preservation Foundation (2010, July 4). Starvation, thirst kill many antelope in Jodhpur. *World Preservation Foundation.* www.worldpreservat ionfoundation.org/blog/news/starvation-thirst-kill-many-antelope-in-jodhp ur/#.UZfB6crHaAY.

Wrangham, R. W. (1974). Artificial feeding of chimpanzees and baboons in their natural habitat. *Animal Behaviour, 22*(1), 83-93.

Ytrehus, B., Bretten, T., Bergsjø, B., & Isaksen, K. (2008). Fatal pneumonia epizootic in musk ox (Ovibos moschatus) in a period of extraordinary weather conditions. *EcoHealth, 5*(2), 213–223.

Zamir, T. (2005) *Ethics and the beast.* Princeton University Press.

(2009). *Ethics and the beast.* Princeton University Press.

Zanette, L. Y., & Clinchy, M. (2020). Ecology and neurobiology of fear in free-living wildlife. *Annual Review of Ecology, Evolution, and Systematics, 51,* 297–318.

Zimmer, C. (2003). *Inside the bizarre world of nature's most dangerous creatures.* Arrow.

Ziomkiewicz, A., Wichary, S., & Jasienska, G. (2019). Cognitive costs of reproduction: Life-history trade-offs explain cognitive decline during pregnancy in women. *Biological Reviews, 94*(3), 1105–1115.

Index

Printed in the United States
by Baker & Taylor Publisher Services